UNDERSTANDING AND TREATING CHRONIC FATIGUE

UNDERSTANDING AND TREATING CHRONIC FATIGUE

A Practical Guide for Patients, Families, and Practitioners

JOEL L. YOUNG, MD

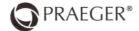

PRAEGER®

An Imprint of ABC-CLIO, LLC

Santa Barbara, California • Denver, Colorado

Library of Congress Cataloging-in-Publication Data

Names: Young, Joel L., author.
Title: Understanding and treating chronic fatigue : a practical guide for
   patients, families, and practitioners / Joel L. Young.
Description: Santa Barbara, California : Praeger, 2020. | Includes bibliographical
   references and index.
Identifiers: LCCN 2020011085 (print) | LCCN 2020011086 (ebook) | ISBN
   9781440871924 (hardcover) | ISBN 9781440871931 (ebook)
Subjects: LCSH: Chronic fatigue syndrome. | Chronic fatigue
   syndrome—Treatment.
Classification: LCC RB150.F37 Y68 2020 (print) | LCC RB150.F37 (ebook) |
   DDC 616/.0478—dc23
LC record available at https://lccn.loc.gov/2020011085
LC ebook record available at https://lccn.loc.gov/2020011086

ISBN: 978-1-4408-7192-4 (print)
     978-1-4408-7193-1 (ebook)

24 23 22 21 20   1 2 3 4 5

This book is also available as an eBook.

Praeger
An Imprint of ABC-CLIO, LLC

ABC-CLIO, LLC
147 Castilian Drive
Santa Barbara, California 93117
www.abc-clio.com

This book is printed on acid-free paper ∞

Manufactured in the United States of America

Contents

Acknowledgments

Writers with an important mission to help suffering people—such as the many who suffer from chronic fatigue syndrome (CFS)—should, in theory, be allotted extra time to practice their craft by the world. But we all receive the same 24 hours to perform daily mundane and major duties as well as achieve long-term goals. This book is the culmination of a significant long-term goal for me. I have had to protect those precious few moments allocated to writing because, as a practicing physician, late evenings and weekends represent the limited time I could carve out for this project. To this end, I am grateful to my wife, Mindy Layne Young, JD, LMSW, who sacrificed much of our precious private time together to allow me to complete my work. My longtime editor, Christine Adamec, structured and paced me, and I deeply appreciate her wisdom and our collaboration. My colleagues at the Rochester Center for Behavioral Medicine provided me with a forum to develop my ideas; I am particularly grateful to Jaime Saal, MA, for her leadership and for guiding our work with Richard Powell, PhD, on the ASSET rating scales. Melissa Oleshansky, PhD, Aliya Pasik, PA-C, and Mavis Emma Buzzard, MA, LPC, generously provided their clinical expertise. I am indebted to Ann Albrecht, Katie Denean, and Didi Nuclej for their daily support over the many years we have worked together. The Clinical Trials Group helped me execute the research that serves at the foundation of this work. I thank my patients for the privilege of being their doctor and for allowing me a position of trust in their lives. This book is dedicated to those who struggle with Chronic Fatigue Syndrome. I have tried to turn your stories into words on a page that can be read and shared with others in the hopes of advancing understanding and limiting future suffering.

Introduction: Overcoming Chronic Fatigue Is Important—and Doable

At my recent medical school reunion, I toasted with the same people I had sat with 35 years earlier. We reminisced about when we clutched our pens while listening to our first lectures on human embryology and when we first cut into the sternum of our willing, forgiving cadaver. In the years since, my lab partner became a noted radiologist, and the president of our class became a superb orthopedic surgeon. One friend has delivered 4,000 babies; another is a top cancer specialist. One of my former classmates chairs a prestigious university's department of internal medicine, but the most important graduate may be the one practicing family medicine alone in a tucked-away small town where medical services are sparse. As for me, I founded and direct the Rochester Center for Behavioral Medicine, a large multidisciplinary mental health clinic outside Detroit, and I serve as the chief medical officer of the Clinical Trials Groups of Southeastern Michigan. In 1985, all my classmates and I were setting out on a long journey, and although we started in the same lecture halls with the same professors, from there our paths diverged. Over time, each found their passion and calling—the development of this book has been my gravitational pull.

Psychiatry is a most fascinating career path; most encounters with patients are intense, and every 30 minutes or so, I can find myself in uncharted territory. During the course of my career, the specialty has also become more powerful—and thanks to innovations in diagnostics and therapeutics, much more can be done for the good of our patients. Although it is true that full cures are elusive, it is rare that contemporary psychiatry is unable to improve the quality of a patient's life.

Individuals with chronic fatigue syndrome (CFS) have proven to be exceptions to this rule. Early in my training, I was drawn to patients who did not quite fit in; and indeed, CFS patients had few places to turn. Their triad of symptoms—persistent fatigue, unexplainable pain, and impaired thinking—are familiar to most primary care doctors, but unfortunately, the medical community has been unable to chart a path forward for those who suffer. Unlike other medical problems, no medical specialty "owns" CFS. A patient with eczema goes to the allergist; a patient with Parkinson's disease sees a neurologist; and if you develop heart disease, you will find care and comfort in a cardiologist's office. In contrast, very few physicians have raised their hands to welcome CFS patients to their practices. Neither did I in the early part of my career, when I knew little about the condition; I proclaimed it not part of my specialty and left the treatment of CFS patients to someone else.

At the beginning of my career, my professional interests lay elsewhere, and I became intrigued by the burgeoning field of attention-deficit hyperactivity disorder (ADHD). I started to care for many adults with ADHD and became deeply familiar with the core treatment for ADHD: long-acting stimulant medications. During this time, I had the revelation that many ADHD patients also complained of persistent fatigue, vague but elusive body pain, and a lack of mental sharpness that we call "brain fog." Quite by chance, I noticed that after treatment with long-acting stimulants, some of these patients reported significant improvement in classic CFS symptoms, such as fatigue and body pain. After several years, I set out to perform a clinical trial comparing lisdexamfetamine (LDX, currently sold under the brand name of Vyvanse) to placebo in subjects with CFS. The results of my double-blind, placebo-controlled study were positive and confirmed my clinical observations. I presented the findings at a national conference and published a formal paper in a peer-reviewed professional journal. The paper drew some interest, but as is my way, I did not shout out my findings from tall buildings to draw in other professionals. I had other tasks to tend to, and I moved on to the next task.

But I did not really move on. In my clinic, I continued to see CFS patients and to spend time learning about their experiences. I became more convinced that CFS is a readily diagnosed syndrome that responds well to available treatments, and I realized I had to amplify my findings beyond readers of scientific papers. CFS wreaks havoc with all in its path; every moment of an individual's life is affected, and they often bear the burden without their family's support or their physician's understanding. CFS has an economic impact as well; the condition negatively affects one's ability to fully produce, and employers lose sympathy with underperforming workers. Insurance companies are reticent to pay disability benefits to clients with a poorly defined disease characterized by invisible symptoms. I am certain that there are many interested parties eager to learn about a viable treatment for CFS and related conditions.

This book is part of a project that has several goals. I am committed to connecting to patients with CFS and related disorders and offering them information about their illness and potential treatment options. I also want to reach out to doctors who work in this field to elaborate a method of approach for this vulnerable population. Finally, I would like to spur a pharmaceutical company that owns the rights to an appropriate medication to scale up a larger, multicenter study to test a thesis proposed in this book: that stimulants often can improve the symptoms of CFS. The CFS community needs and deserves this type of support. Unless I meet these goals, my objectives will not have been fully reached.

All lofty projects need to be grounded in reality. I write this book with the knowledge that I am discussing a class of medications for an indication not approved by the Food and Drug Administration (FDA). I do so in the spirit of sharing an idea and provoking interest. I am most respectful of the need for rigorous scrutiny by others. Note that off-label prescribing is lawful and done frequently by physicians. Doctors can prescribe any approved drug for an indication not covered by the FDA. Of course, physicians should inform patients about both the benefits and the risks of off-label prescribing.

I have divided this book into three major parts. In Part 1, I provide chapters on CFS and explain how this medical problem is differentiated from other conditions, both physical and psychological. I also discuss the theories on the causes of this insidious, life-changing syndrome. In Part 2, I provide a chapter on the Rochester Center's study on CFS, comparing the stimulant LDX to placebo. The following chapter summarizes the various stimulants and "wakefulness" medications that are available today as potential options for clinical application and research exploration. In the last part of the book, I provide a discussion on some of the most troubling symptoms of CFS, including a chapter on how to cope with the overwhelming feelings of fatigue, a separate chapter on how to manage chronic pain, and another chapter exploring the "brain fog" that so many CFS patients encounter. The book concludes with an frank discussion of sleep issues. In my appendixes, I list frequently asked questions (FAQs) as they relate to CFS, a glossary of terms, and screening measures that help physicians assess a patient's issues.

Understanding and Treating Chronic Fatigue: A Practical Guide for Patients, Families, and Practitioners can be read as a whole or as a handy reference. I trust that this guide will help readers better understand this mysterious illness and help them overcome their symptoms with the information I offer.

PART 1

Understanding the Key
Basic Issues

In this part, which includes four chapters, I cover basic but important information about chronic fatigue syndrome (CFS). In Chapter 1, I cover crucial issues, such as who has CFS and why people you know may not understand your symptoms. I also discuss how to explain your illness to others. Chapter 2 covers how CFS is diagnosed, using the "differential diagnosis" process doctors use to consider all possible illnesses and then narrow down to the right one. In Chapter 3, I cover theories about what causes CFS—and there are plenty of them. This chapter is interesting, too, so don't skip it! In the final chapter in Part 1, I discuss other psychological and medical problems that may coexist with CFS, including ones you might expect (like depression and anxiety) and a few you might not have considered (such as restless legs syndrome).

CHAPTER 1

Key Issues You Need to Know about Chronic Fatigue Syndrome

It was only 1:00 p.m., but Diana was so exhausted that she knew she would have to leave work early—again. She had accomplished almost nothing all day, because she just couldn't concentrate. And although she'd achieved very little, Diana felt overwhelmed with exhaustion. Even if she could take a nap here at her busy insurance office—which she could not—she knew that a nap really wouldn't help. When she had tried naps at home on the weekend, she never felt any better when she woke up. Diana thought about having to pick up her children in after-school care and then driving them home and making them dinner—and these tasks felt about as daunting as climbing Mount Everest. What is wrong with me? She wondered. Was it mononucleosis or some sort of major vitamin deficiency? Maybe she needed a complete physical examination. She had to do something, because at this rate, she wouldn't be able to keep her job. Diana didn't know yet that she had chronic fatigue syndrome, a common disorder that she shared with at least 2.5 million Americans nationwide.

If you suffer from chronic fatigue—or CFS—then you are not alone. Millions of Americans stagger around daily like walking zombies from a horror movie because they suffer from chronic pain, difficulty sleeping at night, constant fatigue, and a kind of "brain fog" that feels like being half-alive. If it's CFS, no one knows for sure what causes this medical problem, although I describe every relevant theory I could find in this book. Probably of most importance to my readers is that this book offers real, workable solutions to the problem of chronic fatigue, and I offer individual chapters on how to improve problems like chronic pain, chronic fatigue, brain fog, and sleep disorders. I can't promise to completely alleviate all your chronic fatigue, but I think my solutions can provide real and significant relief.

Why It's Important to Diagnose and Treat CFS

Whether people call it chronic fatigue disorder, myalgic encephalomyelitis/chronic fatigue disorder (ME/CFS), or its newest name (which is quite a mouthful), systemic exertion intolerance disease (SEID), the disorder causing these symptoms can bring strong people to their knees with its symptoms of extreme fatigue, sleep deprivation and unrefreshed sleep, chronic pain, and foggy thinking—none of which is conducive to leading a healthy, normal life. The Centers for Disease Control and Prevention (CDC) says that there are an estimated 2.5 million people in the United States with CFS, and this illness costs the United States up to $59 billion (not million, but billion!) per year in medical bills and lost incomes.[1] That's a staggering amount—and an unsustainable loss to many families.

The disease harms all aspects of a person's life, severely impeding personal, work, and family relationships. But the situation isn't hopeless: treatment can provide major relief to CFS sufferers. If you suffer from CFS, or you know and care about someone else who may have this disease, then the information provided in this book will be meaningful for you. Why? Because there are treatments and therapies that are proven to *work*, and which I hope will also help you. Let's start by explaining what is known about CFS, in terms of the people most likely to develop the disorder.

Women, Men, and Chronic Fatigue Syndrome

Anyone can develop CFS, but some research indicates that females are about three times more likely to develop this disease than are males. In study after study, women have significantly more CFS diagnoses than men. Some research indicates that women with CFS were more likely to have had an early menopause, perhaps prompted by gynecologic surgeries, such as a hysterectomy. Researchers have also found that excessive menstrual bleeding, bleeding between periods, and the presence of endometriosis were also more prevalent in the CFS group compared to the non-CFS group.[1]

However, newer research based on actual diagnostic codes in a large database has indicated that there are more men with CFS than most people realize. In this study, the researchers analyzed data on diagnostic codes based on a database of about 50 million claims for people of all ages over the period 2011–2016. Of all the coded diagnoses, 258,702 people had a diagnosis of either CFS or myalgic encephalomyelitis (both diagnoses are essentially considered the same disease now). The researchers found that up to 40 percent of patients treated for CFS were males.[2]

Why do so many studies indicate that women are the primary CFS sufferers? It's possible that women appear more frequently in many studies of CFS because women may be more likely to volunteer for studies than men. In this diagnostic code study, however, the information was extracted from the computer database, and no human volunteers were needed.

Notes

1. Roumiana S. Boneva, Lin, Jin-Mann S., and Unger, Elizabeth R., "Early Menopause and Other Gynecologic Risk Indicators for Chronic Fatigue Disease in Women," *Menopause* 22, n. 8 (August 2015): 826–834.

2. Ashley R. Valdez, et al., "Estimating Prevalence, Demographics and Costs of ME/CFS Using Large Scale Medical Claims Data and Machine Learning," *Frontiers in Pediatrics* (January 2019), https://www.ncbi.nlm.nih.gov/pmc/articles/PMC6331450/pdf/fped-06-00412.pdf (accessed July 26, 2019).

The Demographics of Chronic Fatigue Syndrome: People Who Are Most Likely to Get CFS

Women are more likely to be diagnosed with CFS than men, although men are also diagnosed with this illness. Other demographic risk factors discussed in this section are intriguing to understand, particularly the age risk, but also others.

Age and CFS

People of any age may develop CFS, but most studies have found individuals ages 30–50 years old are most likely to be diagnosed with CFS. Some studies say that the range is 30–40 years, and others say it's 40–50 years. The Institute of Medicine reports that 33 years is the average age of the first appearance of CFS.[2] It is unknown why people in these age groupings seem to have the preponderance of CFS. It is clear, however, that CFS affects the individual in the heart of life, when their young family relies on them most intensely and when they are trying to move to higher levels in their professional life. Contrast the onset of CFS to that of Alzheimer's disease or even coronary heart disease. These conditions usually present in the later decades of life, and although they cause incalculable suffering, they strike when the patients have already raised their families or completed their careers. Given this delicate time in their lives, individuals with CFS deserve the attention of the medical community.

It's also important to note that some adults with CFS report having suffered from low energy for decades. In addition, keep in mind that children are not immune to CFS (although this book concentrates on adolescents and adults). Parents report that their children with CFS are sluggish and lack the energy that their friends or siblings exhibit. Adults frequently apply very uncomplimentary terms to describe these children. "I have always been told that I am 'lazy and unmotivated,'" a young adult patient with CFS sadly told me. When the symptoms start so early, individuals with CFS can fall behind in their education, their intimate relationships, and their work trajectory. Watching friends and colleagues outpace them is upsetting, but much of the frustration comes from subtle slights. "It hurts to be told that it's all your fault. But if it *is* your fault, then what do you do? How do you make it stop? How do you fix yourself?" The answer is, of course, that it is *not* your fault. This book proposes that CFS is a brain condition–not of your making, not of your choice. And there are actions, discussed throughout the next few chapters that you can undertake to feel better.

Other Demographic Factors

Some studies have found that affluent whites are more likely to develop CFS, while other studies have found the reverse: that low-income minority individuals are at the greatest risk. At this time, not enough is known about racial and socioeconomic factors to conclude which finding is correct. More demographic studies need to be performed to fully describe patients with CFS. From the vantage of my clinic, CFS and related conditions are "equal opportunity diseases" that crosscut many populations. My patients have European, African, and Asian backgrounds. CFS does not discriminate against blacks or whites or Native Americans. Of course, not all Americans have equal access to health care, and part of the motivation of writing this book is to help the CFS population advocate for their own needs in the health care system.

Gulf War Veterans: Chronic Fatigue Syndrome and Fibromyalgia

About 700,000 male and female military veterans served in the Gulf War (1990–1991), and some developed serious service-connected disabilities, including CFS, fibromyalgia, and other health problems. Researchers compared more than a thousand Gulf War veterans to their nondeployed peers, and the researchers found the deployed veterans had a small but higher rate of CFS and fibromyalgia than their peers. For example, 2 percent of the veterans had clinical symptoms of fibromyalgia syndrome compared to 1 percent of the nondeployed veterans. In addition, 1.6 percent of the deployed veterans had CFS compared to less than 1 percent of the nondeployed veterans.[1] No one knows what caused a greater risk for CFS or fibromyalgia in the deployed veterans.

According to the Veterans Administration (VA), military veterans who served in the Gulf War do not have to prove a connection between their service and chronic fatigue syndrome or fibromyalgia, although they do need to receive a diagnosis of one or both diseases to qualify for VA benefits.[2,3] This means that if you have or may have CFS, then you should apply to the VA for assistance. You may wish to ask the American Legion or the Veterans of Foreign Wars (VFW) to help you apply, because the many government forms that are required can be tedious, and it's too easy to make a mistake. In later chapters we will offer some ways to approach your VA doctor about promising treatment for CFS.

Notes

1. Seth A. Eisen, et al. "Gulf War Veterans' Health: Medical Evaluation of a U.S. Cohort," *Annals of Internal Medicine* 41 (2005): 881–890.

2. Veterans Administration, "Chronic Fatigue Syndrome in Gulf War Veterans," December 27, 2017, https://www.publichealth.va.gov/exposures/gulfwar/chronic-fatigue-syndrome.asp (accessed February 13, 2018).

3. Veterans Administration, "Fibromyalgia in Gulf War Veterans," December 27, 2017, https://www.publichealth.va.gov/exposures/gulfwar/fibromyalgia.asp (accessed February 13, 2018).

Chronic Fatigue Syndrome: It Comes with a Price Tag

The CDC estimates that CFS costs the United States up to $37 billion per year in terms of lost productivity. A portion of this sum comprises the direct medical costs of the illness—they may run as high as $14 billion per year.[3] In fact, this could be a low estimate. Earlier in the first decade of the 21st century, researchers analyzed the cost of CFS in the state of Georgia (with a population of about 4 million people). They estimated that the yearly economic costs of CFS for people in this state in the first decade were $1.2 billion in lost productivity and an additional $452 million in health care expenses.[4]

The elegance of the Georgia study design demand that the findings receive a deeper dive into their data. The researchers categorized the 500 subjects into three groups. The first group included individuals who met full criteria for the CFS group. The second group comprised the insufficiently fatigued group (ISF); these were individuals who met at least one criterion for CFS but not all of them. The final group comprised the nonfatigued (NF) individuals. The NF group met none of the criteria and were the healthy control group subjects. This straightforward technique allowed the researchers to fully compare the groups.

The study was well-powered; there were 112 CFS subjects, 264 ISF subjects, and 124 NF subjects. Multiple differences emerged between these three groups. For example, the subjects with CFS earned only about $23,000 per year, and 71 percent of them had been employed in the past four weeks. In contrast, the subjects in the NF group earned nearly $34,000 per year, and 95 percent of them had been employed in the past four weeks. The subjects in the ISF group earned an annual $23,856—not much more than those in the CFS group.[5]

Not surprisingly, the researchers also found that the health care expenditures for the CFS group were significantly higher than for the other two groups; for example, the average health care expenditures for the subjects in the CFS group were $5,683 for the year compared to roughly $3,000 for the ISF group and $2,000 for the NF group. Subjects with CFS had about twice the health care costs of the other two groups.

The researchers concluded:

> CFS attributes to significant economic costs in terms of lost earnings and productivity. Like many other chronic illnesses, productivity loss is even larger than the costs associated with treatment. Such findings suggest that employers are major stakeholders in the search for better diagnosis and appropriate treatment since lost wages are often accompanied by absenteeism costs and health insurance costs that are borne by employers.[6]

Other researchers have analyzed the economic impact of CFS in other areas of the country. A study of patients with CFS in Wichita, Kansas, found a 54 percent drop in terms of labor force productivity tied directly to CFS. The Wichita study estimated that CFS caused a loss of about

$20,000 for each person with the condition. By generalizing this finding to the nation as a whole, the researchers arrived at a figure of a loss of $9 billion per year for all people in the United States with CFS.[7]

No matter who performs the analysis or when the studies are conducted, the costs of CFS to the economy are staggering. The noneconomic costs to the patient, her employer, and her family are even greater.

Coping with Unbelievers within and outside the Family

I think it's important to state here that people with CFS often express dismay that others do not believe that they are truly sick. They don't have a rash, a broken leg, or anything that can be pointed to as the cause of their illness, because CFS is invisible. Even worse, although the CDC, the Social Security Administration, and many other agencies recognize the validity of CFS, many doctors still are dubious that it's a "real" illness, even today. At its worst, the symptoms of CFS affect every moment of every day. The burden is heavier when key members of your life, family, friends, and even your doctors doubt the underlying premise that CFS is a real condition. Too many patients do not receive the validation they deserve.

I believe that the failure to take the condition seriously has two key elements. First, doctors like objective biological signs and quantitative measurements. Medical professionals feel most comfortable when they can visualize a problem through a microscope, endoscope, or a computerized tomography (CT) scan. We know how to measure elevated cholesterol levels and inadequate kidney functioning. We can quickly identify low blood pressure, elevated hemoglobin A1C, and antibodies to the HIV virus. Broken bones appear on the radiologist's screen; calcium deposits are accurately scored by cardiac examinations. Since the 1980s, technology has allowed the profession to quantify considerably more of the human condition than in past years. As with our cars, all this information reduces to flashy dashboards; and health care providers, like the rest of us, are attracted to the method of concentrating information. Quite simply, doctors see abnormal lab values and find reliable ways through medication or surgery to intervene. As there are no clear biological markers for diagnosing CFS, the condition does not fall into this tidy model.

Second, doctors value feeling effective. Addressing a raging infection offers tangible rewards, as does setting a bone, delivering a baby, or lowering someone's ominously high blood pressure. It is far less rewarding to encounter a patient for whom you have little to offer, and it follows that doctors shy away from becoming involved in unwinnable situations. Healers generally do not want to be confronted with a sense of impotency. In many physician circles, treating CFS is seen as fighting the proverbial windmill, and there is often an unconscious (and sometimes deliberate) decision to avoid seeing CFS patients. Many major-referral medical centers in the country will not agree to see CFS patients. In this book we hope to reverse this trend by offering evidence that CFS can be succinctly diagnosed and quantified—and, most importantly, symptoms can respond to specific treatments.

Patients May Feel Like Fakers (And Others May Think They Are Malingerers, Too)

Sometimes, especially if the disease has not been diagnosed yet, people with CFS feel like maybe they really *are* being "lazy" or "crazy" and should just get off their butts and start living again. But when you're in the throes of this illness, the fatigue feels like being submerged in a tar pit. You may have the will of a hero, but your body just will not cooperate.

After talking to hundreds of people with CFS, I developed Table 1.1, a chart of the annoying comments that people with CFS often encounter. I also detail the way many people with CFS respond to the affront. For example, many comments are unappreciated, such as when someone relates that their cousin's wife had that problem and committed suicide. Even supportive comments can be misconstrued; it often seems that no one comes close to understanding your suffering. In the last column, I offer some ways to take the high road whenever possible. However, the barrage of unsolicited comments can be unrelenting—and it's understandable if you slip up now and again.

Beyond the Economic Costs: Other Ways CFS Affects Lives

Some skeptics continue to believe that CFS is a contrived disease, one that was manufactured for lazy people and malingerers to justify their underperformance. Sadly, this stereotype still lingers in the medical community, and this widespread ambivalence creates obstacles to the diagnosis and treatment of this illness. For individuals who are ultimately diagnosed with CFS, it is frequently the case that CFS was not considered as an explanation for five to ten years after their initial complaints.

Even in the absence of good treatment, an accurate diagnosis allows patients to gain a vocabulary to describe their symptoms. For instance,

Table 1.1 Chart of Annoying Comments People Make to Individuals with CFS

Comments People May Make to the Person with CFS	What You May Feel Like Saying	What's Better to Say
Are you sick *again*? When are you going to finally get better?	If I could recover this minute, I would!	Chronic fatigue syndrome is a relapsing disorder, but I'm working on it.
My cousin's wife had that chronic fatigue thing. She killed herself.	So, you think I'm going to kill myself or maybe I should kill myself?	That is very sad, but there is new hope for people with chronic fatigue syndrome.
I wish that *I* could stay home and watch TV all day instead of having to work.	If I could give you this disease for a day, then maybe you would understand it's no fun at all.	I would much rather work and have a normal life than be sick all the time.
I know someone who had that illness, and she began exercising and got all better. Why don't you try working out at the gym?	I can barely get out of bed, and you want me to lift weights and run a treadmill? Are you crazy?	Some researchers have found that active exercise makes chronic fatigue syndrome worse, not better. In contrast, others feel better with physical exertion. It depends on the individual.

postexertional malaise (PEM) denotes the severe exhaustion experienced after physical activity. Yet even this term is deceptive because many individuals with CFS experience fatigue all day long, even in the absence of any exertion. Nonetheless, PEM describes how difficult it is to achieve basic goals of daily life.

The consequences of this illness strongly influence family relationships, work relationships (if the person can continue to work, which often they cannot), and relationships with friends, who may offer various levels of understanding. In this section, I transcribe the words of people who were diagnosed with CFS to convey the effects their illness has had on these relationships, based on their responses to a questionnaire developed by my team and me. Some respondents were recruited on Facebook sites, and others were drawn from my own patient population. All respondents were promised (and given) anonymity.

How Patients Can Explain CFS to Family and Others

Many patients have difficulty explaining to others what CFS is and how it affects them. Keep in mind that dealing with others who question your symptoms often can be frustrating. Table 1.1 illustrates the comments other people may make to you and includes comments you may feel like making and comments we recommend making instead.

Although the listeners may acknowledge the patients are sick, they may believe the doctor should simply give them some medication or treatment that will cure them quickly. Still others will reel off a list of remedies that they think might work, ranging from prescribed drugs to supplements to just-invented devices or other so-called treatments. Here are some facts to help patients explain CFS to their family and others:

- It's a chronic disease.
- You're working on getting help for your symptoms. (Consider sharing those symptoms.)
- You don't know how you got it (unless you think you do).
- It isn't contagious.

Explanation: CFS Is a Chronic Disease

Many people have a simplistic view of diseases. They believe a disease is contracted, similar to strep throat or a urinary tract infection, and that proper treatment will lead to a full recovery. But many diseases are chronic illnesses with no known cure, such as osteoarthritis, heart disease, and high blood pressure (hypertension). There are good treatments for these diseases, and there are also steps that patients themselves can take to improve their condition, such as losing weight, improving their diets, and so forth. However, there is no known cure for many chronic diseases.

CFS is a chronic disease, often with ups and downs that occur for no apparent reason. It parallels allergies in that many patients have periods of intense symptoms and other times of relative calm. Similar to other chronic conditions, such as insulin-dependent diabetes (type 1 diabetes), CFS is not curable. The major thrust of this book, however, is that regardless of whether the FDA has approved a specific medication, effective disease-management options are available. Good treatment of CFS involves an accurate diagnosis, the use of medications, and lifestyle changes—all of which will be discussed in this book.

Explanation: The Patient Is Working on
Addressing Their Symptoms

If you're afflicted with CFS, it's helpful for you to explain to friends, family members, and colleagues that you have sought help for your symptoms. People in your life may not relate to the burden of fatigue, but they can offer needed support. You may encounter some people who do not have the capacity to offer much empathy, and in such cases, sharing your struggle with them can be unproductive. If they are dismissive, then doing so may even be counterproductive.

Your support system will benefit from knowing that the tiredness CFS causes is different from how a person feels after staying up all night and then going to work the next day. Unfortunately, a good night's sleep does not relieve CFS. In fact many people are surprised that daytime symptoms of CFS sometimes may have very little to do with the quality or quantity of nighttime sleep.

Explanation: Patients Don't Know How They Got CFS

Most people have no idea how or why they became afflicted with CFS. Some people have noted that persistent fatigue occurred after a tick bite (Lyme disease) or a bout with mononucleosis or herpes zoster (shingles or chicken pox). Patients may explain that there are many potential causes of CFS, ranging from infectious diseases to injury from a car accident or childhood trauma. Confounding the issue further, not everyone exposed to the Lyme tick, mono, or chicken pox develops CFS. The majority of people with CFS cannot trace their symptoms back to one specific incident. Patients should feel free to divulge if they are unsure how or why they developed CFS.

Explanation: CFS Isn't Contagious

Some things about this mysterious condition are clear. For example, there is no evidence that CFS spreads by air or touch from one human to another or that it is contagious by any other means attributable to being around you. Consequently, there is no reason for people to wear face masks or any other means of protection when they are with you. Even scientists who are convinced that CFS is caused by an infection (a belief not supported in this book) agree that any possible infection preceded the fatigue symptoms by months, maybe years, and that sufferers are not contagious. The bottom line is that humans don't transmit CFS to each other. Many diseases are transmitted human-to-human, but CFS is not one of them.

Why I Wrote This Book

Readers may wonder why a psychiatrist is writing a book on CFS, so it's worth retracing my steps. People suffering from chronic fatigue usually present to their primary care doctor. Sometimes anemia or low thyroid explains symptoms of fatigue, and offering the patient iron supplements or thyroid hormone replacements works well in such cases. However, more times than not, fatigue does not yield to obvious remedies, and after a while, primary care providers refer their CFS patients to various medical specialists in fields such as infectious disease, hematology, rheumatology, and endocrinology. If these long and laborious workups that various specialists may order are not fruitful, often psychiatry is called upon to counsel the patient regarding the frustration of living with a chronic condition. Anxiety and depression are certainly associated with chronic fatigue, but traditionally psychiatrists have been asked to treat these secondary symptoms that result from chronic fatigue rather than to treat the primary symptom of fatigue itself. Psychiatrists concern themselves with the *Diagnostic and Statistical Manual (DSM)*, the professional encyclopedia of mental health disorders. CFS, not considered a mental health condition, is not included in the expansive *DSM*.

Because so many patients with fatigue symptoms have cycled through the existing system without deriving much benefit, and their doctors did not know what else to do, often these patients were sent to me. Early in my career, I would take CFS patients on, and like all the other specialists, I would earnestly try to help them. As I expressed an interest in seeing patients with this presumably untreatable condition, my fellow physicians would express surprise, a touch of sympathy, and a pinch of gratitude.

While the stream of referrals for CFS patients was growing, I was also developing an interest in the treatment of attention deficit hyperactivity disorder (ADHD). ADHD was largely regarded as the province of children, but by the '70s and '80s, psychiatry was starting to explore the natural history of ADHD, and I became intrigued with the question of what ADHD looks like beyond childhood. I became part of the early wave of clinicians willing to treat adolescents and adults with ADHD.

My early years in psychiatry coincided with a dynamic time in ADHD discovery. The most important finding came in a large national study designed to answer the contentious question of the best way to treat childhood ADHD. Some experts believed behavioral therapy was the best approach. Others felt existing medications were superior. The Multimodal Treatment of ADHD (MTA) study demonstrated unequivocally that Ritalin (methylphenidate) played a primary role in ADHD treatment.[8] The MTA study was followed by a serious effort to develop more refined medication approaches, yielding many new ADHD medications beyond Ritalin over the next few years.

Many adults whom I diagnosed with ADHD had initially come to get help for anxiety and depression and had spent many years receiving antidepressant medications. Once they were accurately diagnosed, they benefited greatly from ADHD medications. As I was determined not to miss ADHD, I gave ADHD and other rating scales to all my patients. To my surprise, a few of my CFS patients also met the criteria for ADHD. I eagerly treated them with the appropriate ADHD medication.

I appreciated two meaningful outcomes. First, with treatment, many CFS patients noted improvement in their symptoms. They reported reductions in their inattention and distractibility and improvement in their focus and concentration.

The second finding was less expected. My patients with chronic fatigue began reporting experiencing improved energy. Some announced that they needed fewer naps during the day. They were getting out of bed more easily in the morning. They felt more motivated to get things done. They reported less muscle pain and less reliance on pain medications and physical therapy. Overall, they felt more productive and less overwhelmed.

Why might stimulants work for patients with CFS? Stimulants affect the chemical known as dopamine. Dopamine is present throughout the gut, heart, and brain. When stimulant medications increase dopamine in the prefrontal cortex, several properties emerge. Patients receiving these medications at the right dosage report greater alertness and wakefulness, feeling more activated but not high or altered. The potential utility of these medications in CFS is clear.

A less-understood fact is the property of this class of medications that allows individuals to focus on certain aspects in their environment and filter out other less relevant stimuli. The brain medicated with stimulants filters out the low-level physical symptoms of CFS, such as muscle pain, headache, and achiness. Absent these gnawing symptoms, the patient is better able to find a sense of well-being.

I concluded that long-acting stimulants could play a vital role in aiding the CFS patient.

Overview of Succeeding Chapters

The goal of this book is to develop a guide for the CFS patient and doctor. In the next chapter, I discuss how CFS profoundly affects patients' lives and explore how physicians have regarded CFS over the years. A case study of CFS will illustrate the personal impact of this illness on both the individual and the family.

Chapter 2 provides information on the Institute of Medicine criteria for CFS and the proper approach to considering other explanations for chronic fatigue. The differential diagnosis for CFS is extensive and is essential for doctors to follow to ensure the best outcome for their patients.

In Chapter 3, I will summarize the various ideas proposed over the years to explain the causes of CFS—and there are quite a few theories! Some of these ideas retain strong proponents, some have lost steam over the years, and several have been thoroughly debunked. Nonetheless, readers may be curious to learn about competing explanations for this condition.

Chapter 4 is another important chapter because it covers other diagnoses that commonly appear along with CFS. Patients with CFS may or may not have these diagnoses, but many people do. It's a good idea to treat all of the problems a person may have because even when the CFS symptoms are treated, other problems can impede the patient, including depression, anxiety, fibromyalgia, and other conditions.

I talk about my own research, the Rochester Center Study (RCS), in Chapter 5, and I discuss my success in treating patients with CFS with stimulants. In this chapter, I explain why I performed the RCS, what I found, and the implications of the project. Chapter 6 is a stand-alone chapter with information on long-acting stimulants and how they may play a role in improving CFS symptoms. I also cover the key arguments for and against the use of various stimulant and nonstimulant medications.

Chapters 7–10 are devoted to the core symptoms of CFS, and each chapter provides helpful advice on how to deal with these issues. For example, Chapter 7 covers coping with the severe fatigue that is so characteristic of CFS, including the role of hydrotherapy and other healing modalities. Many people with CFS suffer from chronic pain, and Chapter 8 is devoted to addressing this common problem, whether with nonopioid medications, yoga, or medical marijuana or CBD oil.

Chapter 9 covers what many people call "brain fog," which is a major problem in which the person with CFS becomes aware that she is not thinking well nor is she concentrating effectively or she has become forgetful. No, she doesn't have dementia, although she may fear that she has an early onset of Alzheimer's disease. Useful remedies to combat brain fog are included in this chapter. Finally, Chapter 10 explores the all-important issue of sleep. Many people with CFS get too much sleep because they feel tired all the time, although some people find themselves in bed all day but not necessarily sleeping, and then they experience insomnia at night. This chapter offers practical suggestions to help with sleep problems.

Notes

1. Centers for Disease Control and Prevention, "ME/CFS: Making Strides to Enhance the Lives of Those Living with ME/CFS," May 12, 2017, https://blogs.cdc.gov/publichealthmatters/2017/05/me-cfs/ (accessed February 4, 2018).

2. Committee on the Diagnostic Criteria for Myalgic Encephalomyelitis/Chronic Fatigue Syndrome, Institute of Medicine of the National Academies, *Beyond Myalgic Encephalomyelitis/Chronic Fatigue Syndrome: Redefining an Illness*. Washington, DC: National Academies Press, 2015.

3. Elizabeth R. Unger, et al., "CDC Grand Rounds: Chronic Fatigue Syndrome—Advancing Research and Clinical Education," *Morbidity and Mortality Weekly* 65, n. 50–51 (December 2016): 1434–1438.

4. Jin-Mann S. Lin, et al., "The Economic Impact of Chronic Fatigue Syndrome in Georgia: Direct and Indirect Costs," *Cost Effectiveness and Resource Allocation* 9, n. 1 (2011), https://link.springer.com/content/pdf/10.1186%2F1478-7547-9-1.pdf (accessed March 4, 2019).

5. Ibid.

6. Ibid.

7. Kenneth J. Reynolds, et al., "The Economic Impact of Chronic Fatigue Syndrome," *Cost Effectiveness and Resource Allocation* (2004), https://resource-allocation.biomedcentral.com/track/pdf/10.1186/1478-7547-2-4 (accessed March 8, 2019).

8. The MTA Cooperative Group Multimodal Treatment of Children with ADHD, "A 14-Month Randomized Clinical Trial of Treatment Strategies for Attention Deficit/Hyperactivity Disorder," *Archives of General Psychiatry* 56, n. 12 (December 1999): 1973–1086.

CHAPTER 2

Medically Diagnosing Chronic Fatigue Syndrome

*C*orrie had always been a cautious person and has long maintained a close relationship with her family doctor. She was always up to date with her annual physicals and mammograms. Corrie was a devoted mother of three adult children and was married to Lewis, a recently retired school principal. Corrie remembers her younger self as trying to keep pace with her older but energetic husband. No longer. "For the past several years, my energy is gone, and I feel like a shadow of my former self," she tells her doctor. Tasks that were easy to perform in the past—even getting going in the morning now—take enormous energy. Corrie doesn't know what's wrong with her, but she knows something isn't right. She regularly loses her keys, and last week she forgot to bring in the frozen groceries from the car. Even when she sleeps for 10 hours, Corrie wakes up exhausted.

Although her doctor has sent her to numerous specialists, Corrie wonders again if the doctors have missed an underlying medical condition that explains her fatigue. She asks, "Is this menopause? I have not had a period in five years, so could this be my hormones? Or is this the start of Alzheimer's disease? Is this a sleep disorder? Should I change my diet or exercise more? Which medical specialist should I visit next? How many more tests will be ordered?" Corrie has chronic fatigue syndrome, and what she needs is a careful but not endless medical examination and a definitive treatment plan.

Sometimes—and very distressingly—it takes years for people with CFS to receive an accurate diagnosis, and that means years of frustration and wasted opportunities. It also means meeting with at least a few medical professionals who may wonder aloud if the patient is depressed or has another psychiatric diagnosis. Some sufferers of CFS are accused of "malingering" or just exaggerating their symptoms to avoid work in the pursuit of disability payments.

Corrie doesn't know how to reenergize herself, but if she could do so, she would. She is not depressed. She understands that lethargy and poor motivation can be signs of a biologically based depressive disorder, yet despite her concerns over her chronic fatigue, she does not identify with some of the key components of depression: sadness, pessimism, and suicidal thoughts. Happily married and financially secure, Corrie does not have life circumstances that cause her psychological distress. And like most others with CFS, Corrie really *does* want to work. She has no interest in filing for disability.

Performing a Differential Diagnosis

Doctors are trained to not make snap assumptions about what's wrong with a patient. Thoughtful clinicians will perform a differential diagnosis, which means they will listen carefully to their patient's complaints and consider a whole array of conditions and diseases that might explain the presentation. Corrie's complaints have been long-standing and persistent: chronic fatigue, muscle aches, sleep problems, and a lack of mental clarity so profound that she calls it brain fog.

After considering all possible causes, doctors use their skills of physical examination and understanding of laboratory tests to narrow the diagnosis down to the most likely disease suspects. The ideal physician for the chronically fatigued patient acts like a quarterback—resourceful, encouraging, and always planning the next steps. The examination process for chronic fatigue is extensive, but it needs to be completed in a reasonable period. If the physical examination and lab values are negative—as they often are—then the doctor moves on. She doesn't repeat labs and doesn't send the patient to a specialist unless there is good reason to do so. A prolonged and redundant workup is very stressful for the patient. Sometimes the most honest response a doctor can offer her chronically fatigued patient goes as follows: "I cannot find any medical condition that explains your fatigue. We have ruled out urgent and imminently threatening medical conditions. As CFS is a diagnosis of exclusion, I suspect that is what you have." This decisive language is reassuring to patients with CFS.

Unfortunately, the CFS diagnosis is only half of the work. There are no standard treatment protocols for CFS as there are for other common medical conditions such as asthma or congestive heart disease. It is disappointing to find the proper diagnosis only to learn that dependable treatments are not available. Chapter 1 expands more fully on these issues. Still, I caution the reader that my ideas are novel and have been neither widely adopted nor widely rejected by the medical community. This book and some of my other writings on the topic are intended to bring other clinicians into this important discussion.

This chapter covers diseases that may resemble CFS. These conditions carry universally accepted diagnostic techniques and widely adopted treatments. It is important for the individual with CFS to know what conditions mimic CFS to ensure they are not given a diagnosis that does not fully explain their condition.

Other Conditions That May Mimic Symptoms and Signs of CFS

The very name "chronic fatigue syndrome" demands that the clinician distinguish between long-standing and newly apparent fatigue. Many medical conditions are associated with fatigue, including heart disease, lung disease, kidney failure, infections, malignancies, and other maladies. Overall, these ominous medical conditions yield quickly to routine screening, and physicians can accurately diagnose them early on. For this reason, we do not discuss them further in this chapter. Instead, we focus on other less imminently life-threatening conditions that may mimic CFS. Hypothyroidism, fibromyalgia, Lyme disease, type 2 diabetes, multiple sclerosis, iron deficiency anemia, and vitamin deficiencies such as B12 or magnesium all fall into this category. These disorders are marked by persistent fatigue as well as other symptoms and signs. Comorbid psychiatric diagnoses, which refer to other psychiatric issues often present in people with CFS, are covered further in Chapter 5. For example, in the listless and frustrated patient, major depression is often mistakenly identified as CFS.

Keep in mind that it is possible to have one or more of the disorders covered in this section *and* have CFS, but that is generally unlikely, with some exceptions, such as fibromyalgia. Certainly, if a patient has any of these disorders, treatment will provide improvement to at least some symptoms—and if extreme fatigue continues after treatment, then the doctor can reconsider CFS.

Hypothyroidism

Low levels of circulating thyroid hormone, also known as hypothyroidism, is a common problem in adults. As many as 10 million Americans and up to 10 percent of all adult women are hypothyroid.[1] This condition can cause fatigue and brain fog as well as headaches. Other common symptoms of hypothyroidism include cold intolerance, decreased libido, weight gain, and constipation. Hypothyroidism is readily assessed with a simple blood test, and if the test reveals an out-of-range thyroid finding, supplementation may be needed.

One important point: it is not intuitively obvious, but because of various feedback mechanisms between the thyroid gland and the pituitary gland, higher laboratory levels of thyroid-stimulating hormone (TSH) in tests indicate *low* levels of thyroid. The normal levels on the TSH test range between about 1 mU/L and 2 mU/L, meaning that if a patient's TSH is 9 mU/L, then she is probably hypothyroid. There are some exceptions to this rule—for example, pregnancy can distort the TSH test results, as can serious medical illness. In these circumstances, the doctor may wish to perform a second TSH test before placing the person on thyroid medication. At the other end of the TSH scale, some people are hyperthyroid (with excessively high levels of circulating thyroid hormone). These individuals may exhibit nervous and agitated behavior and usually do not complain of fatigue.

Doctors will want to determine *why* the patient is hypothyroid. The reasons may be related to normal aging rather than to any existing active disease. Most practitioners can readily make this diagnosis and undertake long-term management, but they may look for input from an endocrinologist along the way.

Individuals who are hypothyroid usually respond well to thyroid hormone supplementation, although it may take several weeks to a month before noticeable improvements occur. Clinicians usually start on a low dosage of thyroid medication and gradually increase the dosage based on serial TSH values. This is similar to the way many medications are prescribed. Start low and go slowly.

Fibromyalgia

Fibromyalgia is a common disorder, and understandably, CFS and fibromyalgia are often lumped together. Officially, CFS and fibromyalgia are classified as distinct conditions, yet they share many characteristics. Chronic fatigue is the primary complaint of the CFS patient, whereas pain and stiffness throughout the body characterize fibromyalgia, often affecting the upper neck and back to the greatest extent. As with CFS, people with fibromyalgia often suffer from fatigue and brain fog, but the primary symptom is pain. Complicating the issue further, it is common for a patient to have both CFS and fibromyalgia.

About 4 million adults in the United States have fibromyalgia, and the risk increases with aging. Women are at twice the risk for fibromyalgia compared to men. In addition, people who have had lupus or rheumatoid arthritis have an elevated risk for developing fibromyalgia.[2]

People with fibromyalgia may have difficulty with concentration, memory, and thinking (brain fog), and they may suffer from headaches and sleep problems. Most people with fibromyalgia are diagnosed in their middle age (in their 40s or 50s), although people of any age may be affected by these debilitating symptoms.[3] There are two other distinctions between the two conditions. First, some research supports that physical exercise is helpful for fibromyalgia but may make CFS worse. Second, the FDA has approved several medications to treat fibromyalgia. Pregabalin (Lyrica), duloxetine (Cymbalta), and milnacipran (Savella) all have adequate data studies showing their usefulness for fibromyalgia symptoms. These medications help with certain types of fibromyalgia pain, specifically neuropathy (nerve tingling), and sometimes muscle aching. It is important to note that they do not significantly help with the brain fog, other impairing cognitive symptoms common to fibromyalgia, or CFS. Although this book will explore the utility of stimulant medication for CFS, the FDA has not yet approved any specific stimulant medications for the condition.

Lyme Disease

Every year campers in certain regions of the country are bitten by the tick hosting the *Borrelia burgdorferi* bacterium. This infection can cause Lyme disease, a disorder first identified in Lyme, Connecticut. The tick must remain attached to the person for 36–48 hours to cause infection.[4] At least 30,000 people per year have been infected in the United States, and that number may be 10 times greater, according to the CDC.[5] The Lyme tick is heavily concentrated in the northeastern part of the United States, but people in other parts of the country are infected as well. You can review a map of where the Lyme disease has been identified at this site: https://www.cdc.gov/lyme/datasurveillance/index.html.

The acute symptoms of Lyme disease include fatigue, fever, chills, headache, muscle and joint pain, and swollen lymph nodes. Up to 80 percent of infected people have a rash that looks like a bullseye target, which appears about seven days after the tick bite. The rash may present anywhere on the body.[6]

When Lyme disease is diagnosed in the early stages, the infection can be treated with antibiotics such as doxycycline, amoxicillin, both generic drugs, or cefuroxime (Ceftin). Treatment may last from 10 days to up to three weeks. Most people recover with treatment, but some people develop fatigue and muscle pain that can extend for up to six months.

A more controversial issue is post-treatment Lyme disease syndrome (PTLDS).[7] This diagnosis recognizes patients who have chronic fatigue years after a tick bite. Not all infectious disease doctors agree that the *Borrelia* bacterium can cause long-standing symptoms, and they doubt that it is a valid explanation for chronic fatigue.

In 2012, our team surveyed patients at the Michigan Lyme Disease Conference who self-identified as having PTLDS. A total of 58 adults with PTLDS and a control group of 26 without the condition participated. Surprisingly, most patients surveyed had no recollection of having had an initial tick bite or any acute symptoms. We also found high levels of psychiatric symptoms in the form of anxiety, depression, and ADHD in this group. Of these conditions, depression and ADHD in adults are associated with chronic fatigue. CFS, a condition I have linked to ADHD, may be a better explanation than Lyme disease for the surveyed patients, since it is impossible to have Lyme disease without a history of a tick bite. Additionally, in my clinical experience, the doctors of patients with chronic fatigue migrate to diagnoses that explain the chronic fatigue symptoms via a physical diagnosis such as a post-infectious syndrome.[8, 9]

Diabetes

Patients with diabetes often report feeling fatigued. A diabetic patient told me, "It's like my brain is not working at peak efficiency." Diabetes is a serious disorder of chronically high levels of blood sugar. Often the condition starts in childhood, and patients with insulin-dependent diabetes (type 1 diabetes) must inject themselves with insulin to avoid diabetic ketoacidosis, coma, and death. Type 2 diabetes has a later onset and is often associated with excessive weight. In these cases, insulin may not be needed. A surprising number of people with type 2 diabetes are undiagnosed, which is a tragedy because so many good treatments are available. Patients with type 2 diabetes require careful monitoring of blood sugar levels. Lifestyle changes and medications can extend the quality and duration of life. However, if untreated and/or uncontrolled, there are numerous possible and unpleasant complications, including eye and kidney disease.

A simple finger-prick test may indicate diabetes, but doctors cannot diagnose the disease without a laboratory test known as the HA1c, which reflects blood sugar blood levels for the past three months based on a fasting blood test.

People who are middle-aged and older in their 50s and older and who are overweight or obese are most likely to have type 2 diabetes, although sometimes people with low body mass index (BMI) develop diabetes. Undiagnosed people with diabetes may feel fatigued and constantly thirsty and may need to urinate frequently. Individuals diagnosed with diabetes learn how to control their blood sugar levels with testing. Fortunately, finger-prick tests are becoming obsolete because implantable devices are increasingly available. While type 2 diabetes is distinguishable from CFS, the two are not mutually exclusive conditions. CFS can exist independently along with type 2 diabetes, and CFS should be suspected if fatigue and brain fog continue despite optimal diabetic management.

Multiple Sclerosis

Multiple sclerosis (MS) is a serious chronic inflammatory and neurodegenerative disease characterized by vision loss, pain, fatigue, and impaired coordination. About 400,000 people in the United States have MS.[10] Most (85 percent) MS patients have a relapsing-remitting disease, characterized by feeling worse, then feeling better, then feeling worse again.[11]

MS is more common in women than in men and largely affects white people. In a study of MS in Texas, Missouri, and Ohio, the highest prevalence of MS was found in Ohio, largely among non-Hispanic whites. In another study of more than 24,000 people with MS, the prevalence of the disease was highest among women ages 35–48 and among men ages 40–54. In this study, the prevalence was about three times higher among women than men. The researchers reported the prevalence was higher in the East Census area, which included New England and the Middle Atlantic states, than in other areas of the country.[12]

The most common MS symptom is fatigue, and it presents in up to 80 percent of all affected people. According to the National Multiple Sclerosis Society, MS fatigue can significantly interfere with the person's daily work and other responsibilities. Occupational therapy and physical therapy (PT) may help to combat the fatigue, as may sleep regulation, stress management, and relaxation training.[13] The wakefulness-promoting drug modafinil is often used for MS fatigue. I have found that several of my patients with long-standing MS were misdiagnosed. Inevitably, these patients were diagnosed in an earlier era using indirect diagnostic techniques. In recent years, brain imaging has become more precise, and this diagnostic error occurs less often. It remains good practice to consider MS when a patient presents with fatigue. If, over time, MS symptoms do not progress as might be expected, it is prudent to consider alternative explanations for chronic fatigue, including CFS.

Comparing Well-Being of People with MS and CFS

Most people consider multiple sclerosis (MS) to be a very serious disease—and it is. Yet in a study in the United Kingdom that compared the well-being of patients with MS to those with CFS, the researchers found that the CFS patients were significantly worse off in many respects. This study compared 52 subjects with CFS, 52 with MS, and a third group of healthy controls. The subjects had an average age of 49 years.[1]

The researchers found that 89 percent of the CFS subjects were employed before their illness, but this percentage fell to 35 percent after the onset of the illness. By the time of the study, however, only 13 percent of the CFS subjects were working. In contrast, 93 percent of the subjects with MS worked before their illness, and 60 percent worked after their illness onset. At the time of the study, 37 percent of the MS patients were working. The researchers also found that MS subjects had higher earnings than the CFS subjects. Clearly, the MS subjects, although impeded by their illness, were more able to work than the CFS subjects. The authors poignantly noted that some CFS subjects were only able to continue working "by sacrificing all or much of the social life they would otherwise enjoy."[2]

Notes

1. Caroline C. Kingdon, et al., "Functional Status and Well-Being in People with Myalgic Encephalomyelitis/Chronic Fatigue Syndrome Compared with People with Multiple Sclerosis and Healthy Controls," *PharmacoEconomics Open* 2 (2018): 381–392.

2. Ibid., page 389.

Iron Deficiency Anemia

Individuals with iron deficiency anemia report fatigue and an inability to think clearly. The extent of these symptoms depends on the severity of the anemia. About 10 percent of women of childbearing age in the United States have iron deficiency anemia, primarily from loss of blood with menstruation. Iron-deficiency anemia constitutes about half of all anemias.[14] This disease is diagnosed with a complete blood count (CBC), and patients who have iron-deficiency anemia are treated with iron supplements and other medications.

Common symptoms of iron-deficiency anemia include severe fatigue, pallor, shortness of breath (dyspnea), and the inability to work. Patients who are deficient in iron are given iron supplementation for at least three months.[15]

Other Vitamin and Mineral Deficiencies

Severe fatigue and low energy may be caused by deficiencies in vitamin B12 and by insufficient blood levels of magnesium.

Vitamin B12 Deficiencies

Cobalamin, also known as vitamin B12, is a common blood deficiency and causes fatigue and pallor. Males and females ages 14 years and older need 2.4 mcg of vitamin B12 daily, although pregnant females need 2.6 mcg, and breastfeeding females need 2.8 mcg daily. Vitamin B12 is found in many foods, such as poultry, fish, meat, and dairy products. A B12 deficiency may be treated with injections or oral dosages of this vitamin. Strict vegetarians have an elevated risk for a B12 deficiency, and some drugs may interfere with B12 availability, such as proton pump inhibitors for heartburn, metformin for diabetes, and other drugs.[16]

B12 deficiencies are especially common among people of Northern European ancestry and among older people.[17] It is treated orally or with injections. The method of treatment depend on the severity of the B12 deficiency and the patient's anatomy.

Patients with fatigue due to a vitamin B12 deficiency have a readily addressable medical finding. The medical workup for fatigue should include this simple screening blood test. If supplementation with vitamin B12 does not reverse the fatigue, then CFS should be considered as an alternative explanation.

Low Levels of Magnesium

Fatigue and lack of appetite are early signs of a magnesium deficiency, and if the condition worsens, the person may experience numbness, tingling, and even seizures; abnormal heart rhythms; and muscle contractions and cramps. Those at the highest risk for low levels of magnesium are alcoholics, people with type 2 diabetes, and older adults.[18] Magnesium levels in the blood are easily tested. The doctor may prescribe oral magnesium supplements or, if the condition is severe, she may administer the magnesium intravenously. The average male in the United States ages 31 years and older needs 420 mg of magnesium daily, and the average female of this age needs 320 mg, although pregnant women ages 31–50 need 360 mg daily.[19] It is gratifying for doctors to detect magnesium deficiencies because patients benefit from this simple treatment. If the patient shows little response, do not forget to consider that the true diagnosis may be CFS.

Zeroing In on CFS as *the* Diagnosis

Having ruled out the full possible array of other diseases, the doctor should consider CFS. The Institute of Medicine for CFS revised the criteria for CFS in 2015:

1. A substantial reduction or impairment in the ability to engage in pre-illness levels of occupational, educational, social, or personal activities that persists for more than 6 months and is accompanied by fatigue, which is often profound, is of new or definite onset (not lifelong), is not the result of ongoing excessive exertion, and is not substantially alleviated by rest,
2. Post-exertional malaise,* and
3. Unrefreshing sleep.

At least one of the two following manifestations is also required:

1. Cognitive impairment* or
2. Orthostatic intolerance.
   *Frequency and severity of symptoms should be assessed. The diagnosis of ME/CFS should be questioned if patients do not have these symptoms at least half of the time with moderate, substantial, or severe intensity.[20]

Considering Possible Criteria of CFS

There are five criteria for diagnosing CFS after ruling out other possible disorders, and I discuss each of these criteria in the next sections. In addition, because so many patients with CFS report difficulty with chronic pain, I include a section on this symptom.

Impairments in Social, Educational, Occupational, or Personal Activities

Like all mental health professionals, psychiatrists are accustomed to talking about sensitive issues, past and present, and understanding patients' concerns about troubling aspects of their lives.

To obtain the CFS diagnosis, the patient must have had severe functional impairment at work, at home, at school, or in interpersonal activities for at least six months. Here are some questions that I designed to elicit such information from patients.

1. How well do you think you are doing at work now compared to a year ago? Five years ago?
2. Does it feel like anything is holding you back from performing as well at work as you did in the past? If so, in what ways?
3. Is fatigue a factor in your lower work performance?
4. On a scale of 1 to 10, with 1 being mild and 10 being the most severe, what number would you assign your work performance now?

Post-Exertional Malaise

Postexertional malaise (PEM), a key feature of CFS, describes the severe fatigue and exhaustion that people affected with CFS experience after performing tasks. On some days, tasks as simple as walking the dog or even wiping the kitchen counter can cause this symptom. PEM is diagnosed if an individual regularly overreacts to a mundane exertion. Margot, age 42, has CFS and no other medical condition. One sunny and mild day, Margot's husband encouraged her to join him for a walk in their neighborhood. When she returned 20 minutes later, she fell into a deep sleep in her chair for two hours. "My husband told me that he took my pulse while I was asleep—to make sure I still *had* a pulse!" Margot represents a subgroup of CFS patients who function worse after exercise. For this group, only mild exercise (if any) is recommended.

An event that the individual views as stressful can prompt PEM. As an example, Margot relates that she was mentally and physically exhausted after her eight-year-old child's birthday party. Patients with PEM report that they frequently feel overwhelmed after an event that other people handle in stride. This leads to feelings of fragility and can be a source of contention for family members. Margot lamented, "My husband had to take charge of the party. I am always crashing, and I always feel that I let everyone down."

Many other medical conditions are characterized by fatigue after physical activity; this is the hallmark of various cardiovascular and lung diseases. Doctors don't want to misdiagnose a patient whose post-exertional fatigue is better explained by aortic valve disease or pulmonary fibrosis. The difference is that Margot's fatigue was triggered by mild physical exertion and a routine event such as hosting a child's birthday party. In this way, PEM differs from exercise-induced fatigue.

Postexertional Malaise Is Common with CFS

In a study of 145 people with CFS, researchers found that 90 percent of them experienced postexertional malaise (PEM), not only with physical exercise but also with emotional distress and cognitive exertion (typically worrying about a situation). Eighty-four percent of those with PEM said that this symptom lasted at least 24 hours. Some (11%) said there was about a 24-hour delay between the trigger and the onset of the PEM. Only 9 percent said that the PEM symptoms abated within 24 hours.[1]

In most patients who fatigue with exercise, symptoms begin during the exercise and end soon after exertion stops. This contrasts to the CFS subjects where PEM starts hours or even days after the provocative trigger. In these cases the PEM may last for days, weeks, or even months. Thus, with most subjects, if they feel worse with exertion or emotional distress, they suspend their exercise or remove themselves from the stressful event. People with CFS don't feel worse until much later when the experience is well over, and consequently, they may not make the association between the trigger and the later-occurring PEM symptoms. It is useful for people experiencing PEM symptoms to recollect what they were doing on the day and week before these symptoms took hold. Keeping a diary is a helpful way to identify triggers.

Note

1. Lily Chu, et al., "Deconstructing Post-Exertional Malaise in Myalgic Encephalomyelitis/Chronic Fatigue Syndrome: A Patient-Centered, Cross-Sectional Survey," *PLOS One* (June 1, 2018), https://doi.org/10.1371/journal.pone.0197811 (accessed December 31, 2018).

Unrefreshing Sleep

Another key symptom of CFS is the lack of feeling refreshed after extended sleep. The common problem of nonrestorative sleep is worsened if the patient has trouble falling asleep. Many CFS sufferers report waking up feeling completely unrefreshed after eight–nine hours of sleep. Sleep, a deceivingly complex process of biological renewal, is the key means by which the body repairs itself physically and emotionally and is fundamental to the life process. The combination of insomnia and unrefreshing sleep directly impedes quality of life in patients with CFS.

In the study alluded to earlier by Jain Vageesh, 55 percent of the ME/CFS subjects said they had severe and unrefreshed sleep issues.[21] Many people with CFS have initial insomnia and spend hours trying to fall asleep. Others experience late-night insomnia or awakening before their morning alarms go off. Patients with these problems are also likely to report a diagnosis of obstructive sleep apnea (OSA), a disorder that causes temporary lapses in breathing while asleep. Established treatments for OSA include a continuous positive airway pressure (CPAP) device, a cumbersome bedside device that pumps air into the lung.

Although doctors often order sleep studies for CFS patients, in my experience, the yield is low. In most patients with CFS, sleep studies are negative for OSA. In addition, when using CPAP, many patients have trouble tolerating the inconvenience of sleeping with a face mask. After the long and expensive process of a sleep disorder workup, CFS patients are often left frustrated and with no clear answers.

CFS patients who have insomnia may benefit from cognitive behavioral therapy (CBT) focused on how to develop set sleep routines and to defeat long-standing beliefs that they will never sleep well. At times, sleep-inducing medications are useful, and CFS patients appreciate that their time in bed is spent sleeping rather than rolling around. Unfortunately for many folks with CFS, more hours of sleep do not translate into less daytime fatigue or improved daytime functioning. CFS is more dimensional and extensive than OSA, and the goals of treatment need to include and exceed improving sleep duration and quality. (Chapter 10 expands on the role of sleep in CFS.)

It is essential to understand each individual's specific sleep struggles. The following questions allow the doctor to fully characterize the CFS patient's experience:

1. About how many hours do you sleep at night?
2. Do you have trouble getting to sleep?
3. Do you wake up more than once at night?
4. When you wake up after sleeping at least eight hours, how do you feel, on a scale of 1 to 10, with one being very fatigued and 10 being completely refreshed?

Cognitive Impairment

Cognitive difficulty, also known as brain fog, is another common problem for people with CFS. Patients with brain fog report having regular short-term memory deficits that involve missing an exit while driving on the highway or misplacing their car keys or their wallet. In conversations, they are embarrassed because they forget the names of people they just met and can't access the right words at the proper time. In a study in the United Kingdom of 237 adults with CFS, nearly all subjects reported "trouble concentrating," which was also the most common symptom.[22]

Other cognitive symptoms are difficulty expressing thoughts and slowed thinking. Spouses may lose patience with this absentmindedness and frequently lament that their partners are not listening or staying present in daily conversations. And they're right. Later chapters will provide more information on brain fog.

The following questions can clarify the extent of an individual's cognitive impairment. Keep in mind that most people are overly harsh in their self-assessments and may not accurately remember their earlier effectiveness. These questions are useful only for individuals with mild cognitive impairment and will not yield helpful information when asked to compromised patients with moderate to advanced dementia or Alzheimer's disease. The answers to these questions are more meaningful coming from both the patient and, independently, from their partner or other person who knows the patient well.

1. Do you think you can concentrate as well now as you did in the recent past, such as last year or the year before that? If not, give me an example of better concentration then as compared to now.
2. Are you as good now at making plans and carrying them out as you were in the past? Please explain.
3. If for some reason you had to plan a party or other event, could you do it now? Why or why not?

Other cognitive findings include impaired executive functioning. Individuals with brain fog have trouble planning, sequencing their plans, and motivating themselves to start projects that seem onerous, or they may start projects but not finish them. They might have bursts of curiosity but find it challenging to sustain interest in new things.

Orthostatic Intolerance

Orthostatic intolerance has been associated with CFS/ME (chronic fatigue syndrome/myalgic encephalomyelitis—another name for CFS). A common symptom is feeling faint and dizzy when standing up from a sitting position. Normally, blood pressure rises when people stand, but for those with orthostatic intolerance, blood pressure drops and heart rate increases. Some people with orthostatic intolerance experience blurry vision and see spots in front of their eyes.[23]

In my experience, orthostatic intolerance is a relatively minor finding in a small number of CFS patients. However, there is room for scientific exploration. At a recent National Institute of Health Conference, it was reported that in patients with CFS, prolonged upright posture cause both blood pressure and pulse rates to fluctuate, resulting in an inconsistent blood flow to the brains of CFS patients. The question that emerges from this finding is whether chronic fatigue may result from impaired blood circulation.[24]

The physician should check blood pressure, pulse, and heart rhythm, considering other possible major problems related to heart and vascular disease. In my experience, however, most CFS patients experience these sensations not as the result of fluctuating blood pressure but rather due to their feelings of anxiety and panic. These anxiety symptoms commonly occur with CFS. I discuss other common psychiatric conditions and CFS symptoms in Chapter 4.

A Cautious Word about Orthostatic Intolerance/Postural Tachycardia Syndrome (POTS): What Are They?

Orthostatic intolerance, also known as orthostatic hypotension, has been associated with chronic fatigue syndrome, although this condition is not mandatory for a diagnosis of CFS. Orthostatic hypotension is identified when a person becomes dizzy or even passes out when shifting positions. It happens when a person, usually someone who is older, sits up or stands up too quickly. Usually, upon repositioning, the heart should beat faster, and the arteries carrying blood should constrict to move the blood against gravity into the brain. However, with orthostatic hypotension, faintness occurs when the body cannot quickly and sufficiently accommodate to the new physical position. Though everyone has experienced this sensation on occasion, another related condition, postural tachycardia syndrome (POTS) is diagnosed when this drop in the blood pressure happens repeatedly. Patients with dysautonomia, a dysregulation of the autonomic nervous system, may present with POTS. I have several patients in my practice with POTS who have benefited from medications that control blood pressure or add volume to the blood system.

I have also had patients who have been told that POTS explains their chronic fatigue and brain fog. I believe that this is an inaccurate cause-and-effect explanation, and for that reason, I raise it here. It never made sense to me that this occasional interruption of blood pressure could cause a long-standing effect like brain fog or chronic fatigue. Defenders of the POTS/CFS connection assert that the lower passage of blood through the brain explains chronic fatigue. Linking the conditions appears to be rational but is misleading. Although I have patients whose blood pressure has stabilized on conventional POTS treatments, I have never treated anyone who reported less brain fog subsequent to treatment. Whenever my patients receive the diagnosis of POTS, I usually can find other more feasible explanations for their brain fog and chronic fatigue. Chapters 3 and 4 provide a full discussion into other physical and psychological conditions that mimic CFS and are confused with it.

Chronic Pain

Sadly, most people with CFS report suffering from one or more types of chronic pain. The pain may include muscle aches, headaches, joint pain, and abdominal pain. In addition, the person with CFS may have a chronic sore throat and enlarged and tender lymph nodes. Some female patients with CFS are acutely sensitive to menstrual pain, while others experience pain during intercourse. Men predisposed to pain sensitivity often report constant ear ringing (tinnitus). Added to the burden of enduring these symptoms is that there are often no physical findings. If a broken bone appears in an X-ray or an abscess is red and ugly, no physician doubts the accompanying pain complaints. Conversely, the physical complaint in CFS cannot be visualized, and this frustrates doctors and patients alike. Read more about resolving chronic pain in Chapter 8.

Avoid Opioids for Chronic Pain

It is my clinical experience that CFS individuals treated with stimulant medications experience less pain, and later in the book, I discuss a published clinical trial that supports this observation. Although most of this book offers patients ideas for how to approach their CFS though medication options and lifestyle changes, it is equally important to outline what not to do. Using narcotics (fentanyl, oxycodone, hydrocodone, and so forth) for CFS is misguided and dangerous. Even a brief exposure to opiates can cause tolerance and dependency.

Whereas the first few doses of opioids may relieve pain, ongoing use of opioids makes most CFS patients feel more tired and less mentally aware. Narcotics are not appropriate for most chronic pain conditions, as they are associated with undesirable side effects such as weight gain, temperature intolerance, and constipation. Opioid overdose, a risk that is amplified when combined with other centrally acting medications such as benzodiazepine (Xanax, Klonopin, etc.), is responsible for a great number of deaths every year in our country. Opioids play a vital role in the aftermath of painful surgery and should be available to people with terminal cancer pain, but by every other account, they are the wrong medications for CFS.

Some experts have found that the pain of the person with CFS is significantly greater and/or longer lasting than the pain of healthy individuals who do not have CFS. Severe contrasts emerged in one study of subjects with recently reported pain when comparing subjects with CFS to healthy controls. The researchers found that 73 percent of the CFS patients had muscle pain compared to only 10 percent of the controls, and 64 percent had joint pain compared to 12 percent of controls. (See Table 2.1 for more details.) There are promising means to combat these symptoms, and I discuss these in the treatment chapters, or Chapters 7–10.

After the age of 50 years or so, chronic pain may become a new issue, such as the chronic pain of osteoarthritis, back pain, neck pain, headaches, and so forth. Many people with CFS say that some type of chronic pain is a constant issue in their lives as well. This problem occurs so frequently that, in addition to my individual chapters covering how to cope with chronic fatigue, improve sleep, and manage brain fog (cognitive difficulties), I am including a chapter on dealing with chronic pain. Here are a few simple questions about chronic pain that your doctor may ask you:

1. Do you experience any type of frequent or chronic pain? If so, please describe it.
2. When did this type of pain begin, if you know?
3. On a scale of 1 to 10, with 1 being very mild and 10 being extremely severe, what is the most common rating you would assign to your pain level?
4. What have you done to deal with this pain in the past?

Table 2.1 Comparing Types of Pain of CFS Patients with Non-CFS Patients, by Percentage

	CFS Subjects	Healthy Subjects
Muscle Pain	73 percent	10 percent
Joint Pain	64 percent	12 percent
Headaches	50 percent	7 percent
Tender Lymph Nodes	44 percent	0 percent
Sore Throats	37 percent	1 percent

Source: Leonard A. Jason, et al., "Examining Case Definition Criteria for Chronic Fatigue Syndrome and Myalgic Encephalomyelitis," *Fatigue* 2, no. 1 (January 2014): 40–56. https://www.ncbi.nlm.nih.gov/pmc/articles/PMC3912876/pdf/nihms539096.pdf (accessed July 12, 2019).

This chapter explored the CFS diagnosis and the need to consider other medical problems that might explain fatigue symptoms. It also covered the key features of CFS and explained its primary symptoms, including chronic fatigue (of course). It also introduced other components of CFS, including chronic pain, orthostatic intolerance, and cognitive impairment, commonly referred to as brain fog. The next chapter covers various competing theories regarding the reasons for development of CFS.

Notes

1. James Norman, "Hypothyroidism: Overview, Causes, and Symptoms," *Endocrineweb*, November 27, 2018, https://www.endocrineweb.com/conditions/thyroid/hypothyroidism-too-little-thyroid-hormone (accessed December 28, 2018).

2. Centers for Disease Control and Prevention, "Fibromyalgia," n.d., https://www.cdc.gov/arthritis/basics/fibromyalgia.htm (accessed December 28, 2018).

3. Ibid.

4. National Center for Complementary and Integrative Health, "Lyme Disease," March 2019, https://www.nccih.nih.gov/health/lyme-disease (accessed April 17, 2020).

5. Centers for Disease Control and Prevention, "Data and Surveillance," November 2, 2018, https://www.cdc.gov/lyme/datasurveillance/index.html (accessed December 18, 2018).

6. Centers for Disease Control and Prevention, "Signs and Symptoms of Untreated Lyme Disease," October 26, 2016, https://www.cdc.gov/lyme/signs_symptoms/index.html (accessed December 17, 2018).

7. Centers for Disease Control and Prevention, "Treatment," December 1, 2017, https://www.cdc.gov/lyme/treatment/index.html (accessed December 17, 2018).

8. Joel Young, "ADHD Is Notable Characteristic of Patients Suffering from Chronic Lyme Disease: A Survey of Adults at the Michigan Lyme Disease Association Conference," May 4, 2012, American Psychiatric Association Annual Meeting, Philadelphia, PA, NRD-30, page 212, https://borderlinepersonalitydisorder.org/wp-content/uploads/2012/04/2012_apa_program_guide1.pdf (accessed May 5, 2019).

9. Megan Brooks, "Chronic Lyme Disease Linked to ADHD in Adults," *Medscape Diabetes & Endocrinology*, May 8, 2012, https://www.medscape.com/viewarticle/763458 (accessed July 12, 2019).

10. Piyameth Dilokthornsakul, et al., "Multiple Sclerosis Prevalence in the United States Commercially Insured Population," *Neurology* 86 (March 15, 2016):1014–1021.

11. Curtis W. Noonan, et al., "The Prevalence of Multiple Sclerosis in 3 US Communities," *Preventing Chronic Disease* 7, n. 1 (January 2010), https://www.ncbi.nlm.nih.gov/pmc/articles/PMC2811507/ (accessed December 28, 2018).

12. Piyameth Dilokthornsakul, et al., "Multiple Sclerosis Prevalence in the United States Commercially Insured Population," *Neurology* 86 (March 15, 2016): 1014–1021.

13. National Multiple Sclerosis Society, "Fatigue," n.d., https://www .nationalmssociety.org/Symptoms-Diagnosis/MS-Symptoms/Fatigue (accessed December 17, 2018).

14. M.J. Warner and Kamran, M.T., "Anemia, Iron Deficiency," December 16, 2019, https://www.ncbi.nlm.nih.gov/books/NBK448065/ (accessed March 30, 2020).

15. Ibid.

16. National Institutes of Health, Office of Dietary Supplements, "Vitamin B12: Fact Sheet for Health Professionals," November 29, 2018, https://ods.od.nih.gov/factsheets/vitaminb12-HealthProfessional/ (accessed December 17, 2018).

17. Alex Ankar and Kumar, Anil, "Vitamin B12 Deficiency (Cobalamin)," October 27, 2018, https://www.ncbi.nlm.nih.gov/books/NBK44 1923/ (accessed December 28, 2018).

18. National Institutes of Health, "Magnesium," September 26, 2018, https://ods.od.nih.gov/factsheets/magnesium-HealthProfessional/ (accessed December 26, 2019).

19. Ibid.

20. Committee on the Diagnostic Criteria for Myalgic Encephalomy- elitis/Chronic Fatigue Syndrome; Board on the Health of Select Popula- tions, Institute of Medicine. *Beyond Myalgic Encephalomyelitis/Chronic Fatigue Syndrome: Redefining an Illness*. Washington, DC: National Academies Press, 2015.

21. Vageesh Jain, et al. "Prevalence of and Risk Factors for Severe Cognitive and Sleep Symptoms in ME/CFS and MS," *BMC Neurol- ogy* 17 (2017), https://bmcneurol.biomedcentral.com/articles/10.1186 /s12883-017-0896-0 (accessed February 2, 2018).

22. Ibid.

23. Centers for Disease Control and Prevention, "Primary Symp- toms," n.d., https://www.cdc.gov.me-cfs/symptoms-diagnosis/symptoms .html (accessed December 31, 2018).

24. van Campen, C.M.C., Rowe, P.C., and Visser, F.C., "Blood Volume Status in ME/CFA Correlates with Presence or Absence of Orthostatic Symptoms: Preliminary Results." *Frontiers in Pediatrics* 6 (November 15, 2018), https://www.frontiersin.org/articles/10.3389/fped.2018.00352/full (accessed March 16, 2020).

CHAPTER 3

Theories about the Causes of Chronic Fatigue Syndrome

Traci was finally diagnosed with CFS after 18 months of actively seek-ing a diagnosis for her severe tiredness, chronic pain, and frequent bouts of brain fog. But when she asked the university doctor who had diagnosed her how and why she had developed this problem—what was the cause?—the doctor didn't seem to know how to answer her. Now that Traci had a name for her condition, she decided to search for more answers. Traci uncovered many theories about the causes of CFS, and each one seemed radically different. Some articles asserted CFS was due to an infection, while others said that an autoimmune disorder was responsible. Traci also identified with the theory that CFS was driven by traumatic events; her symptoms started during her parents' divorce and worsened after her second miscarriage. Traci read one article that blamed CFS on people's genes, while her chiropractor told her that fatigue resulted from an overgrowth of gut bacteria. Although Traci was grateful that her new doctor finally gave her condition a name, she was frustrated to not find consensus among experts about what caused her CFS. She wondered why the doctors didn't have this figured out.

Traci is not alone in her frustration; many people with CFS fervently want to understand why they have developed this condition. There have been abundant theories circulated to explain CFS. Some ideas have been announced with great fanfare, while other theories have been proposed and ignored, published in lone journals and now languishing in the dusty stacks of obscurity.

In this chapter, I review some of the common hypotheses advanced over the years about the causes of CFS. Patients with CFS usually visit multiple medical specialists and find that many caring clinicians have tried to understand CFS through the lens of their own discipline. For example, some infectious disease doctors have organized around the belief that CFS results from an infection, although this school disagrees on whether the infection is viral or bacterial. Immunologists and rheumatologists have argued that CFS is an autoimmune disorder, while psychologically based researchers posit that CFS is a reaction to childhood traumas. A controversial specialty, environmental medicine, advances that CFS is a toxic reaction to chemicals in the environment, whereas some women's health advocates led by a group of gynecologists propose that hormonal imbalances explain the problem. This chapter also includes the ideas of some gastroenterologists and geneticists. Ironically, with all of these competing theories spinning about, other doctors dismiss CFS entirely, choosing to believe that if conventional medicine cannot explain it with one unified voice, then it may not be a real disease at all.

A point of order: While there is little consensus about the causes of CFS, it must be recognized as a syndrome, which means it is a constellation of symptoms that all present together. As an example, the syndrome of appendicitis involves the rapid onset of abdominal pain, fever, chills, and nausea. Appendicitis looks the same in Newark as it does in Santa Barbara, and a doctor will spot it quickly whether trained in Beijing or Boston. As young doctors gain clinical experience, they love to exclaim, "Eureka! I have seen this syndrome before, and I know what to do about it." Patients with CFS have a similar presentation that is unique from other conditions. They are "syndromal" because they have a common biological underpinning ensuring that they will have a similar presentation and response to treatment. Although there is no current consensus on what causes CFS, I would love to have a doctor examine a CFS patient after reading this book and declare, "Eureka!" with the same confidence that they bring to other aspects of patient care.

Theory: CFS Was Caused by an Infection

The germ theory of disease is a revered concept, universally accepted by Western medicine. A revolutionary idea when first proposed, the germ theory states that many diseases are caused by microorganisms. A vulnerable host body gets infected by a bacterium or a virus, and a predictable disease follows. Even a child knows the importance of cleaning an open wound lest it become infected with noxious bacteria.

In 1798, Edward Jenner pioneered the concept of vaccination. He inoculated small amounts of cowpox into a young boy, enabling the boy to mount an immune response that ultimately protected him from developing smallpox. More than 150 years later, Drs. Salk and Sabin made similar strides with the polio vaccination. Working under intense pressure, many decades later, virologists determined that the HIV virus was decimating gay men. Because of necessity, researchers developed antiretroviral medications, and public health initiatives surrounding safe sex were introduced. Much of the dying stopped once the germ theory surrounding HIV was deciphered. These and a thousand other stories about infectious diseases have trained doctors to think about disease in this succinct, cause-and-effect manner. When a patient develops a disease, the thinking goes, simply isolate the infectious agent and develop a treatment to contain it or a vaccine to prevent it from ever becoming a threat in the first place.

Unfortunately, applying the germ theory model to CFS has not worked well because CFS has never been proven to be an infectious disease. Yet over the years, doctors and scientists have proposed a number of pathogens to explain CFS. While the evidence does not support this model, it is worth exploring what has been proposed.

Considering the Epstein-Barr Virus

Does CFS develop after an infection? In a study of 535 Australian patients diagnosed with CFS, researchers found that respiratory infections such as colds, influenza, pneumonia, or sinusitis were frequent events prior to the onset of the illness.[1] Several decades ago, Epstein-Barr virus (EBV) was actively considered a cause of CFS. EBV is a prolific virus and is usually the cause of acute infectious mononucleosis. Mononucleosis causes aches, fever, swollen lymph nodes, and an inflamed throat. This infection spreads from person to person via saliva, which is why it is called the kissing disease. It is also spread through sharing the food, drinks, and utensils of those who are infected. EBV can also be contracted through sexual contact or through blood transfusions. Most people completely recover from mononucleosis within a few weeks, although in a minority of patients, stressful circumstances such as going through a divorce or starting basic training can reactivate the infection.[2] A vaccine to prevent EBV is under development.[3]

Although it is clear that EBV is linked to acute mono and occasional reactivation of mono symptoms, some clinicians speculated that the virus might stick around longer, actively triggering aches and fatigue for an extended period. Researchers found that certain patients with CFS had high titers of the EBV antibody. High levels of antibodies usually mean that the antigen, in this case the EBV virus, had infected the body. For many years, some doctors would check EBV titers in their CFS patients and prescribe antiviral medications. Their rationale was that in so doing, they could lower the EBV titers and remove some elements of the disease.

Here is the problem with that logic. It is now known that up to 95 percent of adults worldwide have been infected with EBV[4] and that many folks with and without CFS or a history of mono have had high EBV titers. EBV titers were not unique biological markers for CFS, and therefore nothing could be proven about the hypothesis of EBV triggering CFS. A greater disappointment is that antiviral treatment for EBV did not prove to lessen CFS fatigue. Over time, this seemingly logical idea of EBV causing CFS turned out not to be true. It seemed clear that it was time to move on and rethink the CFS problem.

I include the failed Epstein-Barr (EB) experience for one reason. Years after the EB research was abandoned, CFS patients still ask me to check their EBV titers. They are all disappointed when I tell them there is no reason to draw unnecessary labs because the linking of EBV to CFS did not add up. Some people are so invested in the EB story that they have become angry when I have explained the findings that form my conviction.

These observations have led me to conclude that not only doctors but also many patients in the CFS community are strongly attracted to the germ theory. In their mind's eye, an infectious cause of CFS would give their condition legitimacy. Here's an illness; there's an infectious cause—let's fix it. There is a strong belief that the stigma of CFS would dissipate altogether if an infection were found to cause the condition. Alas, EB infection is not the cause of CFS, but I am sympathetic to the fact that the germ theory is a comforting idea and understand why it is hard to abandon.

Maybe It's a Retrovirus? Oops, False Lead

The EB disappointment did not derail the search for a viral cause of CFS. In 2009, researchers from an Arizona laboratory boldly announced that xenotropic murine leukemia virus-related virus (XMRV), a retrovirus, was *the* cause of CFS. The culprit was at last identified—the condition could be blamed on a particular pathogen. The announcement was heralded in the *New York Times*,[5] and for a brief moment the mystery of CFS appeared to have been solved. The optimism did not last long.

Soon, grumblings about the quality of work in the laboratory surfaced, as did concerns that the researchers had a vested interest in the study outcome. It did not take long for the National Institutes of Health to investigate the lab and determine that XMRV was *not* a pathogen but was instead a human contaminant that was accidentally created in the laboratory. Furthermore, retesting of the blood of patients diagnosed with CFS found *no* XMRV virus whatsoever. The XMRV theory was completely debunked.[6] This notorious case of substandard scientific research was a setback; it increased cynicism in the medical community about the overall legitimacy of CFS, and in the CFS advocacy community, consumers questioned the fundamental motives of once-respected researchers.

Could It Be a Gastrointestinal Infection?

Other microorganisms have been a target for CFS investigation. Giardia is a microscopic parasite that causes the severe diarrheal illness known as giardiasis. In a single study, researchers compared subjects infected with Giardia to healthy controls and found a higher incidence of CFS in the subjects infected with the parasite. Ten years after the infection, 26 percent of the infected subjects had CFS, compared to only 11 percent of the control subjects.[7]

The long-term follow-up of the study was admirable, but the finding does not support the conclusion that Giardia infection explains CFS. We should not forget that, by definition, the fatigue in CFS must come from unexplained etiology, that is, it cannot be better explained by another diagnosis. Having fatigue 10 years after diagnosis is better explained by an insidious parasite depleting the body of essential nutrients than by CFS. This finding would constitute residual chronic fatigue, which is different from CFS. Also, the study was quite small and is now old, and other researchers probably would have tried to replicate the findings had they been intrigued.

Possibly It's a Here Today/Gone Tomorrow Kind of Germ

Other proponents of an infectious cause of CFS assert that CFS could be caused by a hit-and-run type of pathogen, which does its damage and then runs away, leaving no microbial signature. This hit-and-run theory is appealing because it could explain the absence of a biological marker that predicts or measures CFS.

Crime story aficionadas will agree that in the absence of fingerprints, it's hard to retrace a story. Hit-and-run is hard to prove or disprove and highlights the medical community's inability to find a germ theory of CFS. Ultimately, it defies medical logic to support a claim implicating an infection that leaves no biological evidence behind. The bottom line is that CFS may be caused by a virus or bacterium—but if it is, that information is yet unknown. R. A. Underhill summarizes the evidence on CFS as an infectious disease in one statement published in *Medical Hypotheses* in 2015: "No known pathogen has been shown to cause ME/CFS."[8]

Theory: CFS as a Rheumatological or Immune Disorder

Whereas infectious disease doctors question if an infectious virus or bacteria causes CFS, rheumatologists and immunologists wonder if CFS could be linked to an autoimmune disorder in which the body's own defense system attacks itself. A CDC report on CFS indicated that lower levels of natural killer (NK) cells and higher levels of cytokines were found in those infected with CFS. Cytokines are proteins released by the human cells that regulate inflammation. The theory proposes that this impact on the NK cells and cytokines may lead to decreases in the body's ability to respond to physiological stress.[9]

The immune system protects the body by taking defensive actions against invading threats. The immune system can increase the numbers of white blood cells and prompt an inflammatory response to infections and other irritants. Pathogens and other irritants have trouble flourishing when the body's core temperature is elevated, so one form of defense is for the immune system to make the body a less hospitable host through fevers. A prime example of an autoimmune disorder is rheumatoid disease, in which the body attacks itself using many of the defenses listed above.

Could the Cause Be an Immune System in Hyperdrive as a Result of Infection?

Some experts believe that CFS may be caused by an immune system that, for unknown reasons, has begun to overreact to perceived threats to the body. In 2018, a British study fortified this theory. The research centered on 55 patients with hepatitis C (HCV) who were being treated with interferon alpha, a drug that boosts the immune system. Eighteen of the subjects (one-third of the group) developed persistent fatigue.

The researchers found that the blood levels of cytokines markedly increased in the fatigued subjects. In some subjects, these blood levels were more than twice the levels of the treated patients who did not develop persistent fatigue. Cytokines are proteins that the cells release, and some types of cytokines increase inflammation, while others inhibit it. In the study case, the cytokines were the inflammatory types.[10] These kinds of cytokines can cause both fatigue and pain.

According to the CDC, when higher levels of cytokines are present in the body for an extended time, this may lead to the development of health conditions such as CFS.[11] Beyond this theory, there is little clinical evidence that CFS is an inflammatory reaction.

Some Cautions

Two cautions are important for this brief discussion of autoimmune disease and CFS. First, as with infectious disease concepts, immune disorder theories offer an appealing framework for CFS. Autoimmune diseases are rooted in complex science, and CFS is a highly complicated condition. Still, the CDC cautions that research in this field is preliminary and not ready to be applied in patient care. For instance, it is very expensive to test for NK cells and cytokines, and even if they are detected in routine labs, we really do not understand their significance. Just as the infectious disease community could not find an antibiotic or an antiviral to combat CFS, thus far no immunological agents have proven effective in combatting this condition.

My second concern is that rheumatologists, driven by a legitimate interest in helping these patients, may diagnosis CFS patients as having another autoimmune condition and attempt treatment accordingly. This happens when the primary complaint of fatigue co-occurs with diffuse pain or a vague skin rash. From my perch, I have seen CFS patients misdiagnosed as having psoriasis, systemic lupus, or rheumatoid arthritis, even when the clinical picture for these conditions is incomplete. The problem arises when CFS patients are given treatments such as steroids or biological agents for lupus or rheumatoid arthritis (RA). These treatments can be pernicious, and they can lead to long-term complications such as weight gain, a compromised immune system, and even cancer. Furthermore, there is scant evidence that any of these treatments relieves fatigue. Given the potential side effects, it is best not to overtreat CFS patients with immune-based medications.

Renowned Scientist Organizes Colleagues to Understand Son's Severe CFS: Working on a Lab Test for CFS

Ron Davis is a California biochemist and the creator of the nanotechnology that enabled the Human Genome Project to map all human genes. Dr. Davis' son Whitney became ill with CFS in 2011, and he has had a dramatically deteriorating course. Whitney cannot speak or eat solid food, and his parents must provide basic care for their bedbound child.[1]

Dr. Davis and his colleagues are determined to help people like Whitney. Using nanotechnology, the group detected a CFS biomarker, a test to differentiate people with CFS from healthy subjects. Their findings were recently described in the *Proceedings of the National Academy of Sciences*. (For more information, go to https://www.pnas.org/content /pnas/early/2019/04/24/1901274116.full.pdf.) Davis argues that this test might help doctors make an early diagnosis of CFS and differentiate it from other medical conditions. Their work is laborious, and their advances thus far are in the diagnostic, not therapeutic, realm, but hopefully it represents a step forward in CFS research. The CFS community is grateful that a scientist of Dr. Davis's stature is involved in publicizing the plight of patients with CFS and working toward more accurate diagnosis.

Note

1. Ryan Prior, "He Pioneered Technology that Fueled the Human Genome Project. Now His Greatest Challenge Is Curing His Own Son," CNN, https://www.cnn .com/2019/05/12/health/stanford-geneticist-chronic-fatigue-syndrome-trnd /index.html (accessed May 13, 2019).

Theory: Past Abuse and Trauma

Some researchers such as Heim and colleagues[12] have found a correlation between past childhood abuse and the subsequent development of CFS. It is proposed that childhood trauma such as sexual abuse, emotional abuse, or emotional neglect, can cause damage to the brain and body. These repeated psychic injuries evolve into CFS. This theory links a harmful psychic event to a physical outcome and represents a biopsychosocial conceptualization of CFS.

Some CFS sufferers scoff at the link between CFS and early life experiences. After all, the majority of individuals with CFS have not experienced past abuse. They object to the explanation that CFS is the result of psychological trauma, as this implies the need for psychological rather than medical treatment. They object to the suggestion that CFS is in their head and not in their body.

Over the past several decades, medical professionals have become much more attuned to their patients' anxiety and depression. The introduction of Prozac and other serotonin reuptake inhibitors (SRIs) were breakthroughs in the treatment of many mental health complaints. SRIs are now among the most commonly prescribed of all medications, and the public health has benefited from their wide availability and low cost. At the same time, antidepressant medication alone is not sufficient for a patient with an abuse history. Usually, the best approach is to couple medication with psychotherapy; this combination allows patients to have symptomatic relief while giving them the time and space to tell their story. The most effective therapists provide their patients with multiple tools to promote healing.

I am always intrigued by doctors' perceptions of a condition such as CFS, for which clear and effective treatments have not been adopted. On the one hand, lacking a medical explanation, primary care doctors may reason that trauma explains CFS and that mental health professionals are better suited to uncover an abuse history. Alternatively, a doctor may conclude that a CFS patient with an unexplainable problem must be malingering or seeking attention. Doctors are often stymied by their CFS patients. Not knowing how to proceed, they are likely to refer their CFS patients to therapy—sometimes for the right reasons, and sometimes not.

Proceed Cautiously

There are certain problems with linking CFS to trauma or depression. Many individuals exposed to trauma become depressed, yet *they* do not develop chronic fatigue. Often, I have examined CFS patients who have received little or no benefit from repeated treatments of antidepressants. I approach the proposition that psychological trauma causes CFS with the same skepticism that I bring to infectious disease or autoimmune explanations. Having expressed this skepticism, I should emphasize that individuals who have endured childhood trauma typically do benefit from therapy with an experienced therapist. But what about the CFS patient who denies being a victim of past abuse? I suggest that doctors accept this report at face value; these patients should not be referred to therapists who anoint themselves as trauma experts. Too often, these professionals are committed to the notion that the patient with CFS was in fact abused but has not yet come to terms with the experience. The worst of these practitioners impose a narrative on their vulnerable patients, convincing the patients through repetition that there was abuse.

This "recovered memory" approach has flimsy scientific foundation, and if untrue, it can ruin fundamental family relationships. This approach also runs the risk of distracting patients from receiving medical treatments for CFS. (See Chapters 5 and 6.)

I am also skeptical of the practice of reflexively placing CFS patients on antidepressant medications. To be sure, CFS patients with anxiety, depression, and chronic pain may benefit from SRIs or SNRIs. Still, it is important to remember that antidepressant medications are not a comprehensive treatment for CFS. While antidepressant medications combat certain CFS symptoms, they do not address the core complaint of fatigue. In more extreme cases, SRIs are counterproductive; they so deeply mute anxiety that the CFS patient has no motivation at all.

So what is the role of individual counseling in CFS? For CFS patients without a history of abuse, counseling may not be necessary. Conversely, we should refer patients with a history of abuse to therapy, because this form of human connection promotes healing and is an important part of recovery. Counseling in the absence of direct pharmacological treatment, however, is insufficient. Chapter 4 focuses on the psychiatric conditions that are common in patients with CFS and includes an extensive discussion of medication treatment approaches.

Theory: Chemical Sensitivities or Environmental Issues Cause CFS

Another popular and persistent theory is that some people are highly sensitive to the effects of some environmental chemicals and that these toxic elements lead to the development of CFS. Toxic chemicals may include pollutants or heavy metals to which a person is exposed at work, home, or elsewhere. Proponents argue that we are surrounded by unknown toxins and carcinogens. In the 1950s, for example, few people knew that asbestos, an inexpensive insulator, was highly carcinogenic. Of course, asbestos was banned after its link to the fatal lung asbestosis was established. This case and other examples of toxicity have made public health authorities wary of understating other potential environmental threats.

The environmental community has advanced the concept that a subset of individuals develops multiple chemical sensitivity (MCS), an intolerance to substances such as pesticides, smoke, petroleum products, and paint fumes. People with MCS report chronic fatigue, headaches, nausea, and dizziness. Right or wrong, a litany of medical conditions, ranging from Gulf War syndrome to posttraumatic stress disorder, fibromyalgia, and CFS, have been attributed to MCS. As these conditions are not clearly understood and affect thousands of people, including war veterans, some sources, such as the Department of Veterans Affairs (VA), have focused their attention on potential environmental toxins. Faced with mounting suicides, the VA seeks to understand if MCS explains why so many veterans return home with lingering physical and psychological complaints.

Several studies have linked MCS, CFS, and fibromyalgia. Clearly, there is a large overlap in the conditions. A recent study showed that 56 percent of patients with CFS also met the criteria for MCS. Another study showed the rate to be 58 percent.[13] Patients who experienced all three conditions had higher rates of depression and anxiety and lower-quality sleep and social functioning than if they just had CFS alone. High rates of disability were found in this group of patients.[14]

Some MCS advocates link household mold to CFS and have proposed tedious and expensive ways of eliminating all mildew from the home. Other CFS patients have been advised to replace all their old dental fillings.

I have watched patients spend incredible amounts of time and money to comply with these suggestions, desperate to rid themselves of fatigue symptoms (and against my advice). Replacing dental fillings and hiring a mold remediation company may cost thousands of dollars, and sometimes the very expert who advocates the changes is profiting from the person's angst. The theory and practice of MCS can overwhelm a vulnerable patient, who may wonder what else they can do to defend themselves. Should they move to the desert? Isolate their family in the mountains? An overreaction can add to the feelings of isolation and despair that are already too common in those with CFS. How sad and disappointing when even herculean efforts do not resolve their symptoms. There is simply not enough scientific evidence to infer that sensitivity to multiple chemicals is the cause of CFS. Even if MCS does play a causal role, its overall impact is limited, and our search for good answers needs to move in more pragmatic directions.

Theory: It's Hormonal/Gynecological

Women outnumber men in every prevalence survey of CFS, and some experts believe that female hormones are the primary drivers of CFS. They argue that the fluctuating levels of hormones in women of childbearing age trigger the disorder. There is some data to support this idea. In a study that compared 84 women with CFS to 73 healthy controls, researchers found that the women with CFS had a significantly earlier age at menopause onset, or 38 years versus 49 years for the control group. Three-quarters of the women with CFS experienced excessive menstrual bleeding, compared to only 43 percent in the control group. The subjects with CFS were twice as likely to have used noncontraceptive hormonal preparations. As a group, CFS women had a higher risk of pelvic pain, hysterectomy, and other menstrual abnormalities.

So does this mean the problems of CFS women relate to their unstable hormones? This has not been my observation of my CFS patients over the years, and I reject the notion that CFS primarily stems from hormonal fluctuations. Such a theory does not explain CFS in post-menopausal women, and it offers no insight into men with CFS.

Although women with CFS may have more menstrual complaints compared to a control group, pelvic pain and heavy periods do not necessarily cause CFS. Rather, it is my observation that CFS women subjectively experience pain and discomfort more intensely than other women because they have a decreased ability to filter out pain. This is known as hyperalgesia, an increased sensitivity to pain. As a result of hyperalgesia, CFS women are more likely to report painful symptoms and to be offered surgical procedures such as hysterectomies to address these symptoms. The relationship of pain to CFS is covered in Chapters 5 and 8, where I assert that CFS patients treated with long-acting stimulant medications are better able to discern and filter out pain.

Theory: It Was Sedentary Behavior in Childhood

Researchers in the United Kingdom have found a correlation between sedentary behavior in childhood and the development of CFS at age 30. Researchers followed 11,000 children born in 1970 and interviewed them in childhood, adolescence, and near their 30th birthday. They found 93 subjects originally diagnosed with CFS, and 48 currently had the condition. The researchers compared the subjects with CFS to the healthy controls over many different factors, including parental illness, maternal or child psychological distress, academic ability, and sedentary behavior in childhood (defined as only rarely playing sports). The key factor that distinguished the non-CFS group and the CFS group was the sedentary behavior during childhood years. Children who played sports were significantly less likely to develop CFS later in life. Other significant factors were a higher socioeconomic status and physical or mental conditions other than CFS.[15]

It is hard to know how to interpret these findings. Perhaps the sedentary children felt ill and did not have the energy to participate in sports. Perhaps their parents (statistically more likely to have CFS) could not muster the initiative to enroll their children in sports. Or maybe the correlation is accidental and has little or no meaning. An acceptable take-home message for parents hoping to decrease their child's risk of CFS, and for all parents, is to encourage their children to stay active in organized sports.

Theory: Bad Gut Bacteria Did It

Some experts postulate that CFS results from reaction to the wrong type of bacteria present in the digestive system. The theory is that these bacteria subsisting in the small intestine and colon produce toxins that promote fatigue, chronic pain, and sleep problems.

Using sophisticated analyses of bacterial rRNA markers in blood and stool, a group of researchers reported differences between the gut bacteria of subjects with CFS and healthy controls. Bacterial diversity (a wide array of bacteria) was significantly lower in the subjects with CFS than in their healthy cohorts. The researchers also found more bacterial species known to cause inflammation and fewer species that were anti-inflammatory in the subjects with CFS. The theory is that this "dysbiosis" may have triggered an immune response in the subjects with CFS, contributing to the symptoms and severity of CFS.[16]

Again, the cause-and-effect relationship is not clear. Did a certain type of gut bacteria cause the CFS, or did the CFS change the gut composition? It will be interesting to watch the progress in this new area of scientific exploration. As of now, however, these early findings provide little practical application.

Theory: It Could Be Genetic

Some family and twin studies have found links between CFS in children and in their close relatives. There does seem to be a hereditary pattern, but as of now, no candidate genes for CFS have been identified. These are complex determinations to make; people who grow up in the same family are also exposed to the same environmental effects, and this can make it difficult to separate the impact of heredity vs. environment. For example, during childhood and adolescence, they live in the same house, eat many of the same foods, and may share similar habits, both good and bad.

See Table 3.1 for a comparison and brief summary of the pros and cons of the various theories about possible causes of CFS.

Table 3.1 Comparing CFS Theories

Theory of Cause	Pros	Cons
It's a problem with the immune system.	An overworked immune system may lead to CFS.	This theory is hard to prove. There is scant evidence that changing the immune system relieves CFS.
It's viral (or maybe bacterial).	Some evidence points to some viruses, such as the Epstein-Barr virus (EBV) in the development of CFS. A few studies implicate bacteria.	Viruses (and bacteria) are prolific in our society, especially Epstein-Barr virus, but most people with EBV don't get CFS.
It was caused by past trauma or current stress.	Some people with past traumas or high stress levels develop CFS.	Most people with CFS do not report severe past trauma. CFS itself causes stress.
The trigger was a chemical or environmental toxin.	Some people are exposed to toxins including carcinogens, mold, and fumes.	Many people with CFS were not, as far as they know, exposed to chemical toxins.
It's a female problem, related to menstrual difficulties, early menopause, and other related issues.	Some women do experience an increase of fatigue through their cycle and report higher rates of endometriosis, heavy menstrual bleeding, and pelvic pain.	Most women with CFS do not have such problems. Also, postmenopausal women and many men have CFS.
It was sedentary behavior in childhood.	Researchers have found a link between not playing sports in childhood and developing CFS in adulthood.	This could be a correlation without a real meaning, or it could mean that the children had CFS in childhood and did not have the energy to participate in sports.
It's bad gut bacteria.	The "flora" of the gastrointestinal system is important, and can affect how a person feels.	It is unclear if changing the intestinal flora would improve the symptoms of CFS.
It's genetic.	Some twin and family studies indicate a possible genetic connection for CFS.	The gene, if one does cause CFS or otherwise lead to its development, has not been identified. Even if it were identified, it likely would not immediately help people with their symptoms.

What Likely Does *Not* Cause Chronic Fatigue

Most of this chapter concentrates on the many possible causes of CFS, but there are other theories of its causes ranging from unlikely to bizarre that are worth mentioning here. For example, I do not believe that using a cell phone causes CFS (or cancer, or anything else), although if readers are worried about this, then they should use hands-free cell phones or avoid cell phones altogether. Using computers does not lead to CFS— although some people spend far too many hours every day staring at their monitors or laptops, and they need to get up and move around regularly. (That is not exercise; it's basic living.)

There is no need to have all your dental fillings removed because you worry that some substance within them has caused CFS.

Also, as far as I know, neither microwave ovens nor any types of radio waves spark CFS, and childhood immunizations for diseases do not cause CFS.

The Bottom Line

Theories abound on what may cause CFS, whether it is a virus or a bacterium, an overstimulated immune system, a genetic heritability, hormonal factors, environmental or chemical toxins, or stress or past trauma. This chapter has attempted to survey numerous specialties, including infectious disease, immunology, psychology, environmental medicine, gynecology, gastroenterology, and genetics, to ascertain the current understanding that each specialty brings to CFS research. However, the reality is that no one really knows for sure what causes CFS, and although there is some research to suggest that biomarkers will assist in the diagnosis, there is a long way to go in this diagnostic arena as well.

Despite decades of investigation, the cause of CFS remains elusive. It is dispiriting that despite much effort, all we can declare authoritatively is that CFS is an orphan disease. Future research will shed light on the etiology of CFS, but currently, the goal of the physician should be accurate diagnosis, which means excluding those conditions that may look like CFS but are not. Even if the underlying cause remains elusive, it will be prudent to use medications and other strategies that have shown promise.

People with CFS often have other health problems, including anxiety and depression and medical complaints such as tinnitus, interstitial cystitis (IC) (spastic bladder syndrome), and painful muscles and joints. The proper approach to these health problems is the subject of my next chapter.

Notes

1. Samantha C. Johnston, Donald R. Staines, and Sonya M. Marshall-Gradisnik, "Epidemiological Characteristics of Chronic Fatigue Syndrome/Myalgic Encephalomyelitis in Australian Patients," *Clinical Epidemiology* 8 (2016): 97–107.

2. Jonathan R. Kerr, "Epstein-Barr Virus Induced Gene-2 Upregulation Identifies a Particular Subtype of Chronic Fatigue Syndrome/Myalgic Encephalomyelitis," *Frontiers in Pediatrics* 7, n. 59 (March 2019): 1–11, https://www.ncbi.nlm.nih.gov/pmc/articles/PMC6424879/ (accessed May 11, 2019).

3. Gwen Murphy, et al., "Meta-Analysis Shows That Prevalence of Epstein-Barr Virus-Positive Gastric Cancer Differs Based on Sex and Anatomic Location," *Gastroenterology* 137, n. 3 (September 2009): 824–833.

4. K.R.N. Baumforth, et al., "The Epstein-Barr Virus and Its Association with Human Cancers," *Molecular Pathology* 52, n. 6 (December 1999): 307–322.

5. Denise Grady, "Is a Virus the Cause of Fatigue Syndrome?" *New York Times*, October 12, 2009. https://www.nytimes.com/2009/10/13/health/13fatigue.html (accessed October 1, 2019).

6. Hillary Johnson, "Chasing the Shadow Virus," *Discover*, March 27, 2013, http://discovermagazine.com/2013/march/17-shadow-vir (accessed February 21, 2018).

7. S. Litleskare, et al., "Prevalence of Irritable Bowel Syndrome and Chronic Fatigue 10 Years after Giardia Infection," *Clinical Gastroenterology and Hepatology* 16, n. 7 (July 2018): 1064–1082.

8. R.A. Underhill, "Myalgic Encephalomyelitis, Chronic Fatigue Syndrome: An Infectious Disease," *Medical Hypotheses* 85 (2015): 765–773.

9. Alice Russell, et al., "Persistent Fatigue Induced by Interferon-Alpha: A Novel, Inflammation-Based, Proxy Model of Chronic Fatigue Syndrome," *Psychoneuroendocrinology*, December 17, 2018, https://reader.elsevier.com/reader/sd/pii/S0306453018301963 (accessed December 18, 2018).

10. Ibid.

11. Centers for Disease Control and Prevention, "Possible Causes of Myalgic Encephalomyelitis/Chronic Fatigue Syndrome," n.d., https://www.cdc.gov/me-cfs/about/possible-causes.html (accessed May 10, 2019).

12. Christine Heim, et al., "Early Adverse Experience and Risk for Chronic Fatigue Syndrome: Results from a Population-Based Study," *Archives of General Psychiatry* 66, n. 1 (January 2009): 72–80.

13. Alison C. Bested and Marshall, Lynn M., "Review of Myalgic Encephalomyelitis/Chronic Fatigue Syndrome," July 12, 2018, https://www.cdc.gov/me-cfs/about/possible-causes.html (accessed February 4,

2019); An Evidence-Based Approach to Diagnosis and Management by Clinicians," *Reviews on Environmental Health* 30, n. 4 (2015): 223–249.

14. Molly M. Brown and Jason, Leonard A., "Functioning in Individuals with Chronic Fatigue Syndrome: Increased Impairment with Co-Occurring Multiple Chemical Sensitivity and Fibromyalgia," *Dynamic Medicine*, May 31, 2007, https://www.ncbi.nlm.nih.gov/pmc/articles/PMC1890280/pdf/1476-5918-6-6.pdf (accessed May 12, 2019).

15. Russell Viner and Hotopf, Matthew, "Childhood Predictors of Self-Reported Chronic Fatigue Syndrome/Myalgic Encephalomyelitis in Adults: National Birth Cohort Study," *British Medical Journal* (October 6, 2004), https://www.ncbi.nlm.nih.gov/pmc/articles/PMC524102/pdf/bmj32900941.pdf (accessed February 4, 2019).

16. Ludovic Giloteaux, et al., "Reduced Diversity and Altered Composition of the Gut Microbiome in Individuals with Myalgic Encephalomyelitis/Chronic Fatigue Syndrome," *Microbiome* 4 (2016): 4–30.

CHAPTER 4

Chronic Psychological and Medical Conditions That Often Coexist with Chronic Fatigue Syndrome

*R*obert: *I spend a lot of time looking for health information on the internet because I am desperate to feel better! My doctor doesn't know what's wrong with me, and despite all the blood tests and X-rays and CT scans, he still can't figure out what's causing my problems. He probably thinks I'm a raging hypochondriac. But I know what it's like to feel healthy, and it's nothing like this! My wife thinks I'm really uptight and that I spend too much time trying to find something, anything that will explain what's wrong with me! I even thought maybe I had cancer at one point, but no, that wasn't it. Of course I'm glad I don't have cancer, but the NOT knowing why I feel so poorly is so depressing. I read that if there is no other explanation for exhaustion and forgetfulness, I might have chronic fatigue syndrome. I will ask Dr. Brown about it today.*

Dr. Brown: When I see Robert's name on the daily schedule, my heart sinks, and I can't help it. I wonder what disease he thinks he has now. I've ordered plenty of bloodwork, and it all comes back perfectly normal, as did the CT scans. A few months ago, Robert was convinced he had pancreatic cancer, but he had no symptoms and his tests were negative, which I told him. A few weeks later, he was back, and this time he was sure his exhaustion meant he had leukemia. He didn't have that either. His latest idea (probably from Dr. Google) was that maybe he has chronic fatigue syndrome, a disease I'm not sure is even real. I do know that he always seems frustrated and unhappy. I will send Robert to a therapist to treat him for his anxiety.

Dr. Brown had been investigating potential causes of Robert's fatigue for a couple of years. This medical workup (outlined in Chapter 3) was negative. Robert did not have thyroid disease, cancer, anemia, or any rheumatological disease. No overlooked medical illness seemed to explain any of the intermittent symptoms that so frequently brought Robert into the office. Finding no concrete medical answers to explain the fatigue, Dr. Brown seized on Robert's anxious state and referred him for mental health care. Robert left the office feeling defeated and misunderstood.

Robert's case illustrates that often, it is the informed patient who pushes his doctor to consider the possibility of CFS. In fact, most of what Robert learned about CFS came from online searches. CFS is a diagnosis of exclusion, yet even after his full medical work yielded no findings, Dr. Brown did not stop to consider that CFS might be the accurate diagnosis. Rather, the doctor felt stuck and shifted his focus to Robert's anxiety and depression. In so doing, Dr. Brown minimized the debilitating impact of fatigue and signaled to his patient that although he could not offer anything to alleviate the fatigue, emotional support and a gentle antidepressant could help Robert live with the chronic illness. In fact, for most CFS patients, their secondary psychiatric symptoms comprise what others view as their true illness. Like Robert, the majority of CFS patients are diagnosed with an anxiety or depressive disorder—and are treated with anxiety or antidepressant medications. This is generally a positive move; these medications do relieve anxiety and depression.

A more effective treatment directly treats the fatigue. Once the fatigue is addressed, the secondary symptoms of anxiety and depression greatly diminish. Robert is my favorite type of referral because it is so gratifying to offer a new approach to someone who has been written off as a hypochondriac and has lost hope that doctors could help. I receive equal pleasure explaining to my medical colleagues this novel approach to CFS.

This chapter explores health problems that are often present in people with CFS. The first part of this chapter offers an overview of the complex relationship between depression, anxiety, and CFS. These problems often co-occur with CFS and need to be identified and distinguished from CFS. Although CFS is intertwined with these psychiatric symptoms, it needs to be emphasized that the American Psychiatric Association does not list CFS as a psychiatric condition, and there is no psychiatric condition that fully explains CFS.

In the second part of the chapter, I explore common medical problems that frequently appear along with CFS, such as fibromyalgia, migraine headaches, tinnitus, painful bladder syndrome, and myofascial temporomandibular disorder (mTMD). Each of these conditions has unique symptoms, affects different parts of the body, and is addressed by different medical specialties—yet they are strikingly similar in that all these patients complain of persistent and intermittent symptoms and have unremarkable lab values. These conditions are poorly understood, and the failure to treat them results in human suffering and high rates of disability. Using case studies, these conditions are contextualized within the CFS framework, along with the argument that long-acting stimulant medications have a common place in treatment.

Let's start with one of the most prevalent psychiatric problems in the world: Depression.

Depression

Serious depression is a growing problem throughout the world. According to the National Institute of Mental Health (NIMH), in 2017, 17 million Americans adults experienced a major depressive episode.[1] Depression is characterized by feelings of sadness and hopelessness in episodes that last two weeks or longer. The person may also experience fatigue, weight fluctuations, and changes in sleep and appetite patterns. Many depressed patients develop recurrent thoughts of death and suicidal impulses. According to the NIMH, 8.7 percent of American women were clinically depressed in 2017, compared to 5.3 percent of adult males. Women are more likely to reach out for professional help for themselves and on behalf of their family.[2]

Studies have shown depressive disorders are much more common among people diagnosed with CFS than among people with other health problems. For example, a large study compared depressive rates among nearly 23,000 Canadians with cancer, heart disease, and other serious disorders. The disease that won the dubious honor of experiencing the highest prevalence of mood disorders was CFS: 37 percent of CFS patients had mood disorders, followed by nearly 27 percent of patients with fibromyalgia. In contrast, only 10 percent of the patients with cancer were depressed, as were 9 percent of patients with diabetes.[3] (See Table 4.1 for more information). This is an unexpected finding; in my opinion, very few doctors would predict that CFS patients are more likely to be depressed than patients diagnosed with cancer.

Other research confirms and extends this finding. In another Canadian study, 36 percent of 1,045 subjects with CFS were found to have a mood disorder, and nearly one-quarter of these individuals reported that they had considered suicide in the past year. Depressed patients with CFS had many physical concerns. On average, they visited their family doctors 11 times per year, compared to 7.0 visits for the CFS patients who were not depressed. In addition, one in every 11 depressed patients with CFS had seen their family doctor 30 or more times in the previous year.[4] This high utilization rate reveals that while CFS patients are able to gain access to the Canadian health care system, physicians may not be providing them with the right type of relief. No doubt the situation is similar in the United States.

Table 4.1 Prevalence of Mood Disorders in Individuals with Chronic Conditions, Ontario, 2005

Characteristic	Total Number	% with mood disorder
Men	10,105	6.5%
Women	12,528	10.5%
Age group, years		
12 to 29	3,721	8.1%
30 to 49	7,512	10.9%
50 to 69	7,699	8.7%
70+	3,701	4.9%
Married/common-law	14,803	7.6%
Single/Sep/Div/Widowed	7,811	10.8%
Education level:		
Less than second. school	4,975	8.6%
Second. school grad.	3,670	9.1%
Some post-secondary	1,621	10.8%
Post-secondary graduate	11,571	8.4%
Immigrant	6,421	7.2%
Canadian-born	15,500	9.4%
Income within Ontario:		
Low	6,127	11.2%
Middle	7 727	8.6%
High	5,490	6.6%

(continued)

Table 4.1 (*continued*)

Characteristic	Total Number	% with mood disorder
Chronic condition:		
Food allergies	2,108	11.7%
Other allergies	7,636	10.9%
Asthma	3,325	11.4%
Fibromyalgia	637	26.5%
Arthritis/rheumatism	7,140	10.9%
Other back problems	8,089	11.7%
High blood pressure	6,365	8.1%
Migraine headaches	4,721	14.1%
Bronchitis	1,009	16.9%
Diabetes	2,014	9.3%
Epilepsy	215	13.5%
Heart disease	1,997	9.8%
Cancer	621	10.1%
Stomach/intestinal ulcers	1,296	17.0%
Effects of smoke	476	15.5%
Bowel disorder	1,672	17.3%
Cataracts	1,861	8.2%
Glaucoma	610	6.9%
Thyroid conditions	2,183	10.9%
Chronic fatigue syndrome	543	37.2%

Source: T. Gadalla, "Association of Comorbid Mood Disorders and Chronic Illness with Disability and Quality of Life in Ontario, Canada," *Chronic Diseases in Canada* 28, n. 4 (2008): Table 2, page 151, https://www.canada.ca/content/dam/phac-aspc/migration/phac -aspc/publicat/hpcdp-pspmc/28-4/pdf/cdic28-4-4eng.pdf (accessed March 6, 2019). © All rights reserved. *Association of comorbid mood disorders and chronic illness with disability and quality of life in Ontario, Canada.* Public Health Agency of Canada. Adapted and reproduced with permission from the Minister of Health, 2019.

Explaining Depression in CFS

Depression can result from biologic causes, which means that some people are genetically predisposed to developing depression. This means that even in the absence of stressful circumstances, a percentage of the population is at risk of developing depression. It's not uncommon for

me to evaluate a person with a good job, healthy family, and supportive friends who also happens to have an incapacitating depression. In
these predisposed individuals, depression can come unexpectedly, with
no clear triggering event. For others predisposed to depression, everyday
life stress can provoke a new episode of depression. For example, depression can take root when an individual loses a relationship or encounters
a hostile workplace. In a person predisposed to depression, a worsening of CFS or fibromyalgia symptoms can trigger mood symptoms. The
unique suffering of CFS patients is reflected by the fact that CFS patients
report higher levels of depressive disorders than cancer patients. One
reason for this high rate of depression may be that CFS-associated pain
and fatigue feels omnipresent and inescapable. (Note that I have many
suggestions for relief in this book!) Furthermore, cancer patients have
a nonstigmatized diagnosis and a structured treatment plan. Most CFS
patients have neither one.

A positive trend in modern medicine is an increased sensitivity to
a patient's mental health concerns. In previous generations, doctors
did not fully appreciate that treating existing anxiety and depression
greatly improves their patient's quality of life. The introduction of
safe and effective antidepressant medications, coupled with the rise of
patient advocacy movements and changes to federal and state laws in
the last 20 years, have helped to ensure that medical providers screen
for and treat patients with depression. Some major insurance companies measure the rate at which a medical office screens for depression
and uses the data as a quality control measure. If the medical office
does not administer the Patient Health Questionnaire (PHQ-9) routinely
(a simple test for depression), then the doctor's "report card" suffers,
which jeopardizes their per-patient reimbursement. Because of these
types of initiatives, more people than ever are receiving mental health
treatment.

Signs and Symptoms of Depression and CFS Overlap

Table 4.2 compares the symptoms of depression and CFS symptoms.
Note that some of the signs and symptoms of depression sound very
similar to the signs and symptoms of CFS. For example, feeling tired
and unmotivated is common among both groups. Most ratings scales
like the PHQ-9 are not sensitive enough to distinguish between CFS
and depression. This high degree of symptom overlap is why so many
physicians confuse CFS with depression. As a point of distinction, CFS
patients experience more fatigue and pain than depressed patients do.

While depressed patients report that they feel worthless, CFS patients endorse feeling frustrated with their low energy level.

Often, physicians do not distinguish between CFS and depression, and depression becomes the default diagnosis. For this reason, most patients with CFS are prescribed antidepressant medications. Serotonin reuptake inhibitor antidepressants (SRIs) elevate mood, diminish anxiety, and extinguish suicidal thoughts. However, SRIs do not dramatically improve energy or combat brain fog, and it is these cognitive complaints that truly debilitate people with CFS.

Table 4.2 **Comparing Symptoms of Depression and CFS**

Symptom	Depression	CFS
Extreme fatigue	Sometimes	Always; fatigue does not improve with sleep
Lack of motivation to do anything	Sometimes	Common
Feeling like nobody cares about you	Often	Less common
Brain fog	Sometimes	Always or often
Sleeping disturbance	May have insomnia or excessive sleep	Inefficient sleep; time in bed much greater than time sleeping; sleep is not refreshing
Loss of interest in activities that the person used to like	Common. Interest returns as depression lifts	Less common; interested in life activities but has trouble finding energy to actively participate
Depressed mood	Always; sadness is defining feature, and life does not feel worth living Questions the meaning of their existence	Frustrated with their condition rather than feeling hopeless and worthless
Suicidal thoughts	Common	Not typical

Medications and Other Treatments for Depression

Many antidepressant medications effectively treat depression. Patients with CFS who also have depression benefit from these medications. Most increase the concentrations of the neurotransmitter serotonin in the prefrontal cortex and limbic regions of the brain.

First-Line Antidepressants, SRIs, SNRIs, and Trintellix

As mentioned earlier, SRIs are considered the first-line treatment for depression and are widely prescribed. Prozac (fluoxetine) is the most widely known SRI, and there are half dozen others, including Zoloft (sertraline), Paxil (paroxetine), and Lexapro (escitalopram).

A related class of antidepressants are the serotonin norepinephrine uptake inhibitors (SNRI). Some SNRIs are effective for anxiety and diabetic nerve pain, increasing brain concentrations of both serotonin and norepinephrine. The most commonly known medication of this class is duloxetine (Cymbalta). Other SNRIs include venlafaxine (Effexor XR), desvenlafaxine (Pristiq), and levomilnacipran (Fetzima).

Trintellix (vortioxetine) is another type of drug that has a more complicated action mechanism. As with the older medications, Trintellix blocks the reuptake of serotonin, but it also modulates various serotonin receptors. Beyond its effectiveness as an antidepressant for adults, Trintellix has been shown to speed certain cognitive tasks. This property has made Trintellix an appealing antidepressant to use in patients with cognitive deficits such as brain fog.

Antidepressant medications usually take effect within two weeks, and their full effects may not be realized for six weeks. They may cause significant side effects and should not be prescribed casually. Antidepressants are associated with sexual dysfunction and weight gain, and some patients feel emotionally blunted when on antidepressants. It is not uncommon for a patient to report, "Before, I used to cry too easily; now, on medications, I can barely cry at funerals."

Second-Line Medications for Depression

When depressed patients do not respond to first-line antidepressants, antipsychotic medications (Abilify, Rexulti) and mood stabilizing agents (Lamictal) are often added to the SRI or SNRI. In the most severe cases of patients with treatment-resistant depression, Electroconvulsive therapy (ECT) can be administered. The FDA recently approved the antidepressant esketamine (Spravato), a dissociative anesthetic that quickly reverses depression symptoms. Many psychiatrists believe esketamine will prove to be a significant advancement in the treatment of depression and related conditions.

For CFS patients with depression, antidepressant medications are partially helpful. Conversely, a large subgroup of patients with CFS are misdiagnosed with depression and are improperly placed on these medications. Predictably, they do not improve, and unless there is a course correction, they find themselves on increasingly complicated antidepressant medication regimens.

Distinguishing CFS from depression and specifically treating the fatigue and cognitive symptoms of CFS decreases the likelihood of over-treatment with unnecessary medications.

Adjunctive Use of Modafinil (Provigil)

Modafinil (Provigil), a wakefulness-promoting drug, can be added to antidepressant medication in depressed patients with severe tiredness and impaired concentration. Modafinil is a schedule IV drug, and is less regulated than other stimulants (schedule II) because of its low addiction risk. In a study of 60 depressed patients with remitted depression, 30 were treated with modafinil and 30 with a placebo. When comparing the cognition and memory of the subjects in the two groups, the researchers found that the subjects treated with modafinil had significant improvements in the their memory.[5]

In a larger meta-analysis compiling six studies involving 568 patients with major depression and 342 with bipolar depression, modafinil was shown to improve symptoms of fatigue.[6]

In another study, Robert C. Bransfield analyzed 237 patients, with diagnoses ranging from depression to Lyme disease and ADHD. All participants had cognitive complaints, including fatigue, apathy, and concentration impairments. Only a few patients had a sleep disorder. Most of the patients were receiving antidepressants (60 percent) or anticonvulsants (15 percent). Bransfield found that adding modafinil to their baseline treatment improved fatigue, excessive sleepiness, executive dysfunction, and apathy/poor motivation.[7]

Please note that modafinil is not approved by the FDA for depression or for CFS; however, doctors legally may prescribe this drug if they feel it is appropriate. Although technically, it is not a stimulant, modafinil shares certain properties with stimulants. The medication is generally well tolerated but is less effective in CFS than the traditional stimulants I will describe in Chapter 6.

Psychotherapy

For individuals suffering from both CFS and depression, psychotherapy is a meaningful addition to antidepressant medications. A patient's connection to a thoughtful therapist can be powerful. Therapists can explore with clients their feelings about depression, helping them to identify and neutralize negative thought patterns. The therapist can educate her patient that CFS and depression are separate conditions, though often interrelated. She may also educate patients that extended periods of fatigue can give rise to depressive symptoms and that these conditions are rooted biologically. There is no reason for patients to blame themselves for their illness. Therapy involves listening and educating and is most effective in correlation with medication treatment.

Anxiety and Trauma Disorders

Anxiety exacts a heavy toll, and CFS patients are at risk for developing the entire gamut of anxiety disorders, including generalized anxiety disorder (GAD), panic disorder, and post-traumatic stress disorder (PTSD).

Generalized Anxiety Disorders

Generalized anxiety disorder is characterized by excessive worry over a long period. This deeply uncomfortable sensation is accompanied by restlessness, fatigue, impaired concentration, and muscle tension. Individuals with GAD often complain of sleep disturbances and decreased interest in social interactions.

Typically, the GAD patient is consumed with baseless worries about work or the health and well-being of a family member. The patient with GAD has trouble embracing happiness, convinced that good news inevitably will be counterbalanced by something terrible. Everyone encounters transient anxiety on some occasion, but the person with GAD is flooded with persistent worry that lasts at least six months. The anguish is so deep that the person does not gain comfort by a doctor's or friend's reassurance. Women suffer more from GAD than men, with 3.4 percent of all women affected compared to 1.9 percent of men.[8]

Certain behavioral patterns occur in GAD:

- Worried thoughts in a loop (thinking the same worries, over and over)
- Feeling that something *must* be done—but not knowing what to do or how to get started
- Worry that they will cause problems for other people in their life
- Fears about personal safety and the well-being of friends and family

Becca, a human resources manager with GAD, described the endless loop of her intimate thoughts.

I know I *have* to solve the staffing problem at work, but I don't know what more to do. I've tried everything that I can think of, but nothing has worked so far. If I do not solve the problem, I could lose my job! Then we won't have any money to pay the bills, and I'll probably lose my house and our health insurance. I can't tell my boss that I'm stumped because when I do turn to him, he doesn't make me feel better. He would probably fire me. I must solve this problem, but I don't know how! What the heck am I going to do? I must do something, but what?

Becca displays a thought process of "catastrophizing," believing that the worst possible outcome will happen. While she knows intellectually that her boss has no intention of firing her and that the company's current staffing problems are manageable, she finds little comfort in these facts. While Becca welcomes reassurance from others, the relief does not last long, and the worry quickly resurfaces. GAD is addressable with medications and therapy.

Panic Attacks

Panic attacks come out of nowhere. Within minutes of its onset, the patient develops heart palpitations, sweating, shortness of breath, trembling and shaking, chills, and hot flashes. Along with these physical symptoms, an impending sense of doom engulfs the patient. The fear of dying is overwhelming, and a high percentage of people experiencing their first panic attack end up in the hospital emergency room, certain they are having a heart attack or stroke.

Panic attacks usually dissipate as quickly as they appear, but sometimes the patient starts to fear that the attack will recur. The experience is so unpleasant that sufferers modify their lives to decrease the likelihood of having another panic attack. Patients develop avoidances; for instance, if they had a panic attack on the freeway, then they avoid the freeway or avoid driving altogether. If the panic attack occurred at the supermarket, they may avoid the store or refuse to shop alone.

Post-traumatic stress disorder can develop when an individual is exposed to overwhelming events such as combat or a natural disaster. Post-traumatic stress disorder can also emanate from abusive experiences in childhood or a physical or sexual assault. Some of the symptoms closely resemble those of GAD and panic disorder, but PTSD patients uniquely experience an altered sensation of reality, referred to as dissociation, as well as an inescapable feeling that they are constantly reliving the trauma.

The Link between CFS and Anxiety

It is important to unravel why CFS patients are more likely than others to have anxiety. People with CFS seem to overreact to their environment and feel unduly threatened. Panic symptoms then follow.

While they are no more likely to experience a hurricane or a robbery than the average person, they may have a harder time calming themselves in the aftermath of a threatening event, and this increases their likelihood of developing PTSD. In other parts of the book, I assert that many adults with CFS also have lifelong ADHD, a condition that starts in childhood. Children and adults with ADHD are more likely than others to have experienced traumatic experiences. For example, in a study of 216 adults with ADHD compared to 123 adults who did not have ADHD, 10 percent of the adults with ADHD had PTSD, compared to about 2 percent of the controls.[9]

Another factor contributing to anxiety is that CFS patients may be accused of malingering, or faking their illness. Others may believe they are lazy or deluding themselves into thinking they are sick in order to gain sympathy. Some people with CFS have been suspected of gaming the system to receive disability payments or even to create an excuse for their tepid performance at work or home. The burden of feeling exhausted and in pain is hard enough, but feeling invalidated and manipulative compounds the discomfort.

It may also be that people with chronic fatigue too successfully hide their symptoms and how they feel about them. There is also experimental evidence that CFS patients may process emotions differently than others, specifically by suppressing their underlying feelings. In a study of 80 adults with CFS and 80 healthy controls, researchers exposed all subjects to an upsetting movie clip. Half of each group were told to suppress their feelings, while the other half was encouraged to express their feelings as they wished. Electrodes placed on the skin measured the subjects' physiological responses to the movie clip. Third-party observers were told to report levels of distress among the subjects. Based on their skin measurements, the CFS subjects had significantly *more* distress than the healthy controls; however, the observers perceived *low* levels of distress in the CFS subjects. To clarify, the CFS subjects were actually quite upset based on their physiological responses, but they did not *seem* upset to others. The researchers questioned whether this disparity accounts for CFS patients being less able to utilize social supports during periods of stress.[10]

Although the study concludes that CFS patients process emotions differently from normal controls, it still does not answer the pivotal question: does CFS cause anxiety, or does early-life trauma trigger fatigue?

Somatic Symptoms Disorder, Anxiety, and Chronic Fatigue Syndrome

Patients with CFS are especially susceptible to somatic anxiety, or excessive worrying about one's health. In a British study of 45 patients with CFS, including 31 women and 14 men, the researchers administered the Short Health Anxiety Inventory and the Hospital Anxiety and Depression Scale. They found that 42 percent of the subjects had significantly elevated levels of health anxiety. This far exceeded the rate of health anxiety found in patients with other health issues.[1]

It is interesting to speculate as to why this happens. The authors of the study conclude that patients with CFS feel "delegitimized" by their symptoms, and this leads to uncontrollable anxiety. This, along with their misperceptions of symptoms, the tendency to catastrophize, and the proclivity to feel overwhelmed offers sober explanation. Patients with CFS resent their fatigue and grow endlessly frustrated by not having good treatments or explanations.

There is some good news to counter these sober observations. When I have used stimulant medication to treat CFS, the anxiety symptoms decreased. This is contrary to what most people would predict, but in a double-blind study of lisdexamphetamine (LDX) versus placebo in the CFS patients, their anxiety scales declined significantly with active treatment. Clinically, I have found that treated patients become less preoccupied with anxiety and health concerns. The medication appears to allow them to "filter out" distractions, which allows them to process baseless worries into more productive thoughts. With long-acting stimulant medications, the patient's compulsion to visit the doctor for every health concern diminishes. Chapter 5 explores this study in depth.

Note

1. Jo Daniels, Brigden, Amberly, and Kacorova, Adela, "Anxiety and Depression in Chronic Fatigue Syndrome/Myalgic Encephalomyelitis (CFS/ME): Examining the Incidence of Health Anxiety in CFS/ME," *Psychology and Psychotherapy: Theory, Research and Practice* (2017), https://onlinelibrary.wiley.com/doi/abs/10.1111/papt.12118 (accessed February 1, 2019).

Other Medical Problems That May Coexist with CFS

Patients with CFS frequently present with nebulous medical conditions that interfere with their quality of life. Many of these conditions are poorly understood, and while some treatments are available, the response to treatment is highly variable. I will discuss five of these interrelated conditions: fibromyalgia, chronic headaches, painful bladder (also known as interstitial cystitis), ear ringing (tinnitus) and mTMD.

Each condition affects a different region of the body and the attention of a different medical specialist. For instance, neurologists quarterback headaches, urologists handle bladder concerns, and ENTs and dentists examine patients with tinnitus and jaw pain. Because these conditions are dispersed among medical specialists, and as fatigue complaints are overlooked, it is challenging to draw common conclusions about these disparate medical problems, but I will try to do so.

Several features are common to all these complaints. First, they are all associated with chronic fatigue. Second, the examining doctor often cannot find an anatomical reason for the complaints. Finally, the symptoms arise, dissipate, and arise again over time. Most importantly, I have found that in the presence of chronic fatigue, treatment with long-acting stimulant medications forces many of the physical symptoms into retreat. Let's discuss each with greater detail and an anecdote of a successful treatment outcome in each case.

Fibromyalgia

The muscular aches and pains of fibromyalgia are commonly seen in outpatient clinics. Fibromyalgia often occurs in people with CFS, and many clinicians lump the two medical conditions together as one entity. Although they can occur together, fibromyalgia and CFS are officially distinct ailments. Fibromyalgia is characterized by occasional fatigue and so-called tender points, along with migrating pain through the body. Conversely, some pain might be reported with CFS, but the fatigue is the defining feature. According to the CDC, fibromyalgia affects an estimated four million people in the United States.[11]

Common symptoms of fibromyalgia include the following:

- Stiffness and pain throughout the body
- Sleep problems
- Fatigue and tiredness
- Struggles with memory and concentration
- Frequent headaches, such as migraines[12]

Other symptoms may include the following:

- Muscle fatigue and cramps
- Irritable bowel syndrome

- Painful menstrual periods
- Temperature sensitivity
- Depression or anxiety[13]

Fibromyalgia is most common among middle-aged individuals, although the disorder can occur in people of any age. Women are about twice as likely as men to have fibromyalgia.[14] Other factors linked to fibromyalgia include obesity and past injuries.

Treatment for Fibromyalgia

In the past decade, three medications have been developed for fibromyalgia, while CFS remains an orphan illness, with no single medication yet approved. Duloxetine (Cymbalta) is an SNRI approved by the FDA for the treatment of fibromyalgia, as is a related drug, milnacipran (Savella) that is less popular. Pregabalin (Lyrica), which is not an antidepressant, can also be used to treat diabetic nerve pain. Patients with fibromyalgia may also receive both prescribed and over-the-counter anti-inflammatory medications and pain control agents. Opioids should be avoided for this chronic condition.

Physical therapy is a mainstay of fibromyalgia treatment. Exercise is also recommended, although some research suggests that for those who have both fibromyalgia and CFS, exercise may worsen symptoms. Cognitive-behavioral therapy may play a productive role, and stress-management techniques such as yoga, meditation, and acupuncture may help certain patients, at least in the short term.

Headaches

Headache pain is associated with tension in the neck, shoulders, and crown of the skull. Frequent headaches may be linked to stressful circumstances and elicited by certain foods.[15] Migraines are a specific type of headache characterized by an aura (seeing flashing lights or smelling something that is not there) prior to the onset of the actual headache. Chronic migraines are headaches occurring at least 15 days each month, and they affect about 1 percent of the population, according to the American Migraine Foundation.[16]

Risk factors for chronic migraines include the presence of other pain disorders, the presence of a back or neck injury, and obesity. Migraine rates are higher in those with a diagnosis of anxiety and/or depression.[17] Often, migraine sufferers endure both classic migraine and tension headaches.

Success rates of treatment vary widely. Medications may include over-the-counter drugs, such as acetaminophen or ibuprofen. Prescribed medications are primarily in the triptan category, such as sumatriptan (Imitrex) and rizatriptan (Maxalt), among others. Botox injections are also increasingly common treatments. In addition, biofeedback and relaxation therapy may both be helpful techniques for migraine sufferers.

Because my colleagues know I have an interest in the underpinnings of chronic medical conditions, I have often been asked to evaluate patients who seek help for headache and migraine. One of my patients was Cary, a 47-year-old engineer. Cary had chronic fatigue and migraines and had been on triptans and Botox injections. Of concern was that he had used opiate medications for years, and his new doctor did not want to continue his prescription.

After a formal evaluation, I diagnosed Cary with ADHD, predominantly inattentive type, and with CFS, and his prescription was Adderall XR twice daily, a standard treatment for ADHD. I fully expected his inattentive symptoms to improve, and they did. An added benefit was the reduction in his profound fatigue. An unexpected byproduct of the Adderall XR treatment was a decrease in the frequency and intensity of his headaches. Cary now uses triptans (migraine medications) rarely, and he also discontinued the expensive Botox injections. Both Cary and his internist are delighted that he no longer needs opioid analgesic medications.

Other researchers have explored the connection of migraine to CFS. In one study, 82 percent of subjects with CFS experienced migraines, compared to 13 percent of healthy controls.[18] If the hypothesis that CFS responds to long-acting stimulants proves valid, then it might also represent a plausible treatment for chronic migraine. It is also worth noting that caffeine, a stimulant, has long been added to headache medications, including the iconic brand Excedrin. Complicated patients such as Cary, who have migraines, CFS, and ADHD, may benefit from further research.

Painful Bladder Syndrome (Interstitial Cystitis)

Painful bladder syndrome is a chronic condition experienced by up to eight million people in the United States, primarily females. Whereas the average woman urinates four to seven times per day, women with painful bladder syndrome may have the urge 40 times a day. Other symptoms may include pain during sexual intercourse and pain in the lower back or abdomen that escalates during the menstrual period.[19]

Initially, the presentation of severe bladder pain may point to a bladder infection, but the urinalysis and culture are both negative. This problem can be further analyzed with a cystoscopy, or an internal examination of the bladder by a urologist. Other tests may include a biopsy of the bladder to check for bladder cancer. With the patient under sedation, the urologist may fill the bladder with fluid to stretch it and to determine how much fluid the bladder can hold. During this procedure, the urologist may or may not find lesions on the bladder wall.

Urologists have difficulty understanding why some women have excruciating bladder pain in the absence of lesions, and others have lesions but no pain. This does not mean the pain is not real in some people, but the intermittent nature of the complaints is mysterious. It is noted that IC often runs with other chronic health problems such as CFS and fibromyalgia.

Traditional treatment for painful bladder syndrome often does not work dependably because the underlying cause is unclear. Proposed treatments may include over-the-counter painkillers or prescription medications such as pentosan (Elmiron). Antihistamines and/or antidepressants may help, as might Botox injections. Surgery to clear the lesions has not been widely adopted. Women are advised to stop smoking and to avoid citrus fruits, alcohol, tomatoes, and chocolate—all foods that can irritate the bladder.[20]

Interstitial cystitis (IC) patients come to my clinic because they are frustrated with their unrelenting pain. My patient Ellie had all the symptoms of IC, painful bladder syndrome. Despite close adherence to her treatment plan, including taking scheduled pain medications and limiting her diet, she still had persistent bladder pain. Our evaluation determined that in addition to anxiety, Ellie also had ADHD, predominantly inattentive type, and CFS. I added Vyvanse to her long-standing antidepressant medication.

My primary goal was that the medication help Ellie focus and concentrate, and she did appreciate relief quickly. She also noticed a lessening of her bladder pain. Over time, Ellie reported that she used her IC medications less often. Her urge to void decreased, and intercourse became less painful.

When I questioned Ellie, she emphasized that the pain was not gone, but she felt less preoccupied by the sensation of bladder discomfort. The discomfort was more evident in the morning before she took her Vyvanse and in the evening after the medication wore off. On the days that Ellie did not take Vyvanse, her pain resurfaced. I concluded that not only did Vyvanse enhance her attention but it also distracted her from the unpleasant physical sensation emanating from her bladder. This helps explain the intermittent nature of physical complaints; whether the pain comes from a lesion or another source, the brain has the ability to filter out irritating signals. Medications such as Vyvanse can temporarily district the brain from registering the discomfort.

Ringing in the Ears (Tinnitus)

Not a day goes by in an ENT's office when a patient does not complain of tinnitus. The description of the sound varies—a ringing or crackling in the ears; sometimes constant and other times intermittent. The sound may be a clicking or hissing type of noise, and it may be either low-pitched or high-pitched. There are some known causes of tinnitus, such as a noise-induced hearing loss and ear or sinus infections. Many can empathize with tinnitus sufferers; indeed about 10 percent of American adults have experienced at least five minutes of tinnitus in the past year.[21] For those who experience tinnitus chronically, the problem can lead to impaired quality of life and debility.

Causes of Tinnitus Are Unclear

Scientists disagree on why people develop chronic tinnitus; it may stem from damage to the inner ear's signaling action in part of the brain. People with chronic tinnitus may gain some relief through wearable or tabletop sound generators, which help drown out the internal noises that the person constantly hears. For those who have experienced hearing loss along with their tinnitus, hearing aids may help. More sophisticated and elaborate treatments include acoustic neural stimulation with headphones and a handheld device that sends a broadband acoustic signal embedded in music. This treatment may desensitize the person to the tinnitus, and it has been effective in volunteer testers.[22]

As the referral activity between otolaryngologists and psychiatrists is minimal, I assume I see only a smattering of tinnitus patients. My impression, however, is that currently available treatment is often ineffective. The strategy of mechanically distracting the patient with other sounds does not consistently work. Because effective treatments are elusive, tinnitus patients are a great source of frustration for their doctors. In kind, tinnitus patients express their dissatisfaction for the care they receive.

The Case of Barry

Barry suffers from tinnitus. His ear ringing began after he sat under the speakers at a loud concert in an enclosed room. "Several times that night, the high-pitched feedback from the speaker jarred me," he said. In the succeeding weeks, Barry was so impaired that he could not go to work. He was a dedicated triathlete, and to make matters worse, a recent tear to his Achilles tendon dropped his exercise to nothing. Barry became irritable, and his relationship with his family and work colleagues deteriorated. Over the next few months, he saw two ENT physicians, and over the next year, he tried many different treatments. He attended his son's wedding wearing noise-cancelling headphones—but received more odd stares than relief.

Barry was disturbed to learn that a prestigious clinic refused to see him, stating that they had nothing more to offer for his tinnitus. He came to me to seek help regarding his fatigue, poor motivation, and family conflict. Barry's wife bitterly complained of his compulsive need to exercise for up to six hours per day, an unexpected behavior in a man suffering from fatigue. During Barry's evaluation, I learned that two of his children had long been treated for ADHD. When asked, he reported that he had always been fidgety. "That's why I always exercise. If I don't move, I feel like crawling out of my skin." Barry's diagnosis was clear: ADHD, hyperactive-impulsive type.

I started Barry on Mydayis, a stimulant medication, and he engaged in talk therapy. Within a few weeks, many of his complaints lifted, and his ear ringing reemerged only in emotionally stressful circumstances. Mydayis arrived in Barry's life in time to salvage his job, and he was able to avoid filing for disability insurance. Barry realized that since starting treatment, he felt calmer, and upon recovery from surgery, he no longer craved endless exercise. A 45-minute workout three or four times weekly was sufficient.

Myofascial Temporomandibular Disorder (mTMD)

Myofascial temporomandibular disorder (mTMD) is a common type of temporomandibular disorder. The temporomandibular joint includes the bones, muscles, and tissues forming the area between the upper and lower jaw. Clinical signs of mTMD include muscle tenderness upon pressure to the joint or surrounding area, causing restrictions on movements of the mouth. The patient may notice clicking noises when opening and closing the jaw.[23] This medical problem is associated with pain upon awakening, muscle tenderness, and severe migraine or tension headaches. Often the pain comes on suddenly, rather than increasing slowly over a period. Nearly half of all patients with oral and facial pain have mTMD.[24]

Before making the diagnosis, the doctor should rule out other conditions that can cause facial pain. These include dental cavities, a cracked tooth, sinusitis, and irritation of the trigeminal nerve in the cheekbone area (trigeminal neuralgia).[25]

Dentists are usually the ones who treat mTMD. Dental appliances can be fitted and are often used in tandem with naproxen (Naprosyn) or another nonsteroidal anti-inflammatory drug (NSAID). Injections of local anesthetic is a more invasive approach. Other drugs that may be employed are anticonvulsant medications such as gabapentin (Neurontin) and pregabalin (Lyrica) and a tricyclic antidepressant—most often amitriptyline (Elavil). Benzodiazepines medications such as diazepam (Valium) and clonazepam (Klonopin) may help combat muscle tension in the short term, but they have fallen out of favor due to the potential for addiction and the risk of severe complications when used with muscle relaxants such as cyclobenzaprine (Flexeril) and opiate medications.[26]

Because traditional treatments for mTMD are problematic, many doctors refer patients to PT. If PT fails, alternative treatments such as acupuncture or biofeedback therapy remain. Biofeedback therapy teaches the patient to relax when pulse or blood pressure increase during pain. Some patients obtain short-term relief from these approaches, but they rarely work over a longer period.

Wrapping It Up

Although mTMD, chronic migraine, IC, and tinnitus all affect different parts of the body, they share common features: waxing and waning pain complaints, often with no corresponding physical finding for the pain. Most of them, certainly mTMD, present commonly among people with fibromyalgia and/or CFS.[27]

Other medical maladies too numerous to detail also fall under this general description. They include irritable bowel syndrome (IBS), some aspects of premenstrual syndrome (late luteal dysphoric disorder), lower back pain, and a controversial condition called postural orthostatic tachycardia syndrome (POTS). There are clear causes for some cases of these conditions, but for many patients, there is no answer. The treatments that do exist help select patient but not others. Sometimes patients gain hope when a specialist appears, offering a new approach, and lose hope after she leaves, mission not accomplished. Even well-meaning and enthusiastic doctors must move on—leaving their patients feeling abandoned.

In my experience among the heterogenous conditions discussed in this chapter, CFS is often a common denominator. Modulating central dopamine channels with long-acting stimulant medication alleviates fatigue and allows the brain to filter out painful stimuli. Further research in the use of this class of medications holds promise for many of the patients discussed in this chapter.

This chapter covered other issues that people with chronic fatigue commonly experience, ranging from depression and anxiety to health problems such as fibromyalgia, tinnitus, and other issues.

In the next chapter, I dig deeper into my own research and describe the findings of the RCS, which compared a long-acting stimulant to placebo in a CFS population. I follow this with a discussion of the types of medications that may be helpful in making a meaningful difference in the lives of people with chronic fatigue.

Notes

1. National Institute of Mental Health, "Major Depression," November 2017, https://www.nimh.nih.gov/health/statistics/major-depression .shtml (accessed February 1, 2019).

2. Ibid.

3. T. Gadalla, "Association of Comorbid Mood Disorders and Chronic Illness with Disability and Quality of Life in Ontario, Canada," *Chronic Diseases in Canada* 28, n. 4 (2008): 148–154.

4. Esme Fuller-Thomson and Nimigon, Jodie, "Factors Associated with Depression among Individuals with Chronic Fatigue Syndrome: Findings from a Nationally Representative Study," *Family Practice Advance Access* (October 2008), https://academic.oup.com/fampra /article/25/6/414/480969 (accessed February 8, 2019).

5. Muzaffer Kaser, et al., "Modafinil Improves Episodic Memory and Working Memory Cognition in Patients with Remitted Depression: A Double-Blind, Randomized, Placebo-Controlled Study," *Biological Psychiatry: Cognitive Neuroscience and Neuroimaging* 2, n. 2 (2017): 115–122.

6. Alexander J. Goss, et al., "Modafinil Augmentation Therapy in Unipolar and Bipolar Depression: A Systematic Review and Meta-Analysis of Randomized Controlled Trials," *Journal of Clinical Psychiatry* 74, n. 11 (November 2013): 1101–1107.

7. Robert C. Bransfield, "Potential Uses of Modafinil in Psychiatric Disorders," *Journal of Applied Research* 4, n. 1 (2004): 198–207.

8. National Institute of Mental Health, "Generalized Anxiety Disorder," November 2017, https://www.nimh.nih.gov/health/statistics /generalized-anxiety-disorder.shtml (accessed February 1, 2019).

9. Kevin M. Antshel, et al., "Posttraumatic Stress Disorder in Adult Attention-Deficit/Hyperactivity Disorder: Clinical Features and Familial Transmission," *Journal of Clinical Psychiatry* 74, n. 3 (2013): e197–e204.

10. Katharine A. Rimes, et al., "Emotional Suppression in Chronic Fatigue Syndrome: Experimental Study," *Health Psychology* 35, n. 9 (2016): 979–986.

11. Centers for Disease Control and Prevention, "Fibromyalgia," October 11, 2017, https://www.cdc.gov/arthritis/basics/fibromyalgia.htm (accessed February 1, 2019).

12. Ibid.

13. Office on Women's Health, "Fibromyalgia," August 22, 2017, https://www.womenshealth.gov/files/documents/fact-sheet-fibromyalgia .pdf (accessed February 7, 2019).

14. Ibid.

15. Joseph Kandel and Sudderth, David, *The Headache Cure: How to Uncover What's Really Causing Your Pain and Find Lasting Relief.* New York: McGraw-Hill, 2006.

16. American Migraine Foundation, "Chronic Migraine," May 2008, https://americanmigrainefoundation.org/resource-library/chronic -migraine/ (accessed February 1, 2019).

17. Ibid.

18. National Headache Foundation, "Illness, Chronic Fatigue Syndrome and Migraine," March 15, 2013, https://headaches.org/2013/09 /15/illness-chronic-fatigue-syndrome-and-migraine/ (accessed February 7, 2019).

19. Office on Women's Health, "Bladder Pain," December 27, 2018, https://www.womenshealth.gov/a-z-topics/bladder-pain (accessed February 7, 2019).

20. Ibid.

21. National Institute on Deafness and Other Communications Disorders, "Tinnitus," March 6, 2017, https://www.nidcd.nih.gov/health /tinnitus (accessed February 7, 2019).

22. Ibid.

23. Robert L. Gauer and Semidey, Michael J., "Diagnosis and Treatment of Temporomandibular Disorders," *American Family Physician* 91, n. 6 (May 15, 2015): 378–386.

24. César Fernandez-de-las Penas and Svensson, Peter, "Myofascial Temporomandibular Disorder, *Current Rheumatology Reviews* 12, n. 1 (2016): 40–54.

25. Robert L. Gauer and Semidey, Michael J., "Diagnosis and Treatment of Temporomandibular Disorders," *American Family Physician* 91, n. 6 (May 15, 2015): 378–386.

26. Ibid.

27. No author, "Options and Perceptions: Rethinking Treatment for Facial Pain," *Pain Week*, February 5, 2019, https://www.painweek.org /media/news/options-and-perceptions-rethinking-treatment-facial-pain (accessed February 7, 2019).

PART 2

Learning How
Medications May Help

In this part, which includes two chapters, I talk about my own research study of the use of stimulants with people with chronic fatigue in Chapter 5, and then in Chapter 6, I discuss stimulant medications in general that may be used to improve the symptoms of a person with CFS.

CHAPTER 5

The Rochester Center Study on Stimulants and Chronic Fatigue

When he returned to his hometown to practice psychiatry after completing his residency training, Dr. Y was greeted with a large caseload. His colleagues learned that the young doctor was interested in treating patients who had not fared well with their current treatments. Dr. Y also expressed an interest in adult ADHD, a niche that was basically unfilled. Referrals were directed in, and the psychiatrist scrambled to find his stride. He was clear what to do for patients with anxiety, depression, and ADHD but was less sure how to approach patients who were concerned about their generalized fatigue and chronic pain.

In his psychiatric residency training, scant attention was given to patients with fatigue and chronic pain. He was taught the standard medical workup for fatigue but noticed in nearly all of these patients that the usual suspects (thyroid abnormalities, anemia, or underlying cancer) did not explain the fatigue. While the doctor was struggling to develop a meaningful intervention for his chronically fatigued patients, his other patients—notably, those with adult ADHD—were flourishing. Dr. Y noticed that some of his ADHD patients also complained of chronic pain and fatigue, and he observed that treatment with standard ADHD medications, specifically stimulant medications, significantly relieved their fatigue symptoms. On these medications, patients reported more energy and less pain; their need to visit the chiropractor or physical therapist diminished; and most importantly, they were able to back off their opiate pain medications. In case after case, Dr. Y made this same *observation, and he became eager to share these findings with other colleagues.*

As you may have guessed, I am the "Dr. Y" in the opening anecdote, and since this book has many stories about people, I indulged in writing one about myself. For many years, I discussed my observations about chronic fatigue in informal discussions with fellow doctors and published several case studies for wider distribution. I soon realized that for any new idea to gain traction, it must be scientifically proven. A formal clinical study is the best way to confirm or refute a new treatment. Meaningful studies are double blind and placebo-controlled and are structured so that patients with CFS are randomly assigned into one of two groups. One group receives the active agent, and the other group receives a sugar pill. Neither group knows which group they are assigned to because they receive identical-looking capsules. My hypothesis was that in a study population of CFS, patients given the long-acting stimulant medication LDX (Vyvanse) would have greater improvement in cognition, fatigue, and pain complaints compared to subjects given placebo.

Of course, when a clinical study is performed, one can never be certain of the outcome. Science and medicine are full of stories in which ideas were dismissed after negative results from a double-blind, placebo-controlled study. In this case, I only wanted to know the truth—I had no vested interest in proving the hypothesis, I owned none of the rights to the medications, and I had nothing to gain from a positive study. What truly motivated me was advancing a treatment option for people with chronic fatigue and related conditions.

In this chapter, I will describe the Rochester Center Study (RCS), comparing LDX to placebo in patients with chronic fatigue who are experiencing executive function deficits. Spoiler alert: the study revealed that LDX *did* improve cognitive function and other symptoms commonly known as brain fog. When compared to placebo, LDX also improved symptoms of pain, anxiety, and fatigue. The implication of the study for CFS and many of the medical and psychiatric conditions associated with CFS are discussed. The chapter concludes with a case study of Abby, a patient who waited years to get diagnosed with CFS but who greatly benefited from LDX.

Background of the Rochester Center Study on Chronic Fatigue

I have spent the past 25 years as medical director of the Rochester Center for Behavioral Management (RCBM) in Rochester Hills, Michigan. RCBM is an outpatient psychiatric clinic staffed with psychiatrists, psychologists, psychiatric nurse practitioners, physician assistants, mental health counselors, and social workers. We are a team of 60 professionals with a single mission of tending to the mental health needs of our patients. Working parallel to RCBM is the Clinical Trials Group (CTG) of Southeastern Michigan, where I serve as chief medical officer. For over 20 years, CTG has participated in clinical trial research; in this capacity, we are approached to conduct national clinical trials of a new medication or of an existing medication that needs to undergo further testing. I have been the principal investigator in more than 90 clinical trials. CTG has studied scores of different medications, ranging from antidepressants to antipsychotics to psychostimulants. We have studied numerous clinical conditions, including eating disorders, treatment-resistant depression, bipolar disorder, and movement disorders. Many of the medications now approved by the FDA and widely prescribed were at one point studied at CTG. Not everything we studied has gone on to be a successful medication. More than once, I received urgent calls instructing me to immediately suspend an ongoing clinical trial because an early analysis of the data found the medication unsafe or ineffective. In clinical research, there are good days and bad days.

At RCBM, we treat patients ranging from ages 4 to 100. At CTG, we have studied preschool tic disorder, eating disorders in adolescents, and late-life dementia. Still, not all research questions are of equal interest. A respected pathologist once confided to a group of medical students, "You will find over time that each of you has your favorite disease." This is a complicated statement to unravel because, as doctors, we must be the enemy of all disease. In medical school and training, we all learn about the entire spectrum of human illness, but in practicality, we can only become experts in a few.

Early in my career, I observed the link between treatment with stimulants and CFS, but it was a decade or so later, after I had additional clinical research experience, that I felt ready to organize a clinical trial to explore whether this observation held up under closer scrutiny. The burning question I needed to resolve was this: Do psychostimulants improve cognition in patients with CFS? And if so, what other aspects of CFS do they improve? Most importantly, are they safe to use in this population?

Undertaking the Project

Many elements are necessary to conduct a research study, and trials involving human subjects are complicated and expensive to pull off. All clinical trials require a protocol, which are the rules governing each step of a trial. This protocol went through many revisions and was reviewed by many experts; a statistician determined that if our single site could obtain data on 26 subjects, the study would have enough statistical power to draw meaningful conclusions.

The next challenge was to obtain approval from an Institutional Review Board (IRB). Decades ago, research on human subjects was performed without close oversight, and this led to unethical conditions that were unfair to study participants. Contemporary standards demand that study participants be fully aware of the process and give their informed consent. We approached the Western Institutional Review Board, an established IRB, to review our proposal. They scrutinized our protocol, made some changes, and ultimately approved our study design. CTG took all measures to ensure that our research protocol was carefully executed and ensured the safety of our subjects.

We also needed to find a sponsor to fund the study and supply the study drug. I was interested in studying LDX, which is a prodrug compound developed by Shire Pharmaceutical, allowing for a long-acting effect over time. At the time, LDX was newly approved for ADHD. Shire offered support for investigator-initiated studies and agreed to supply us with the LDX capsule and look-alike placebo capsules. The company had no say in the protocol or in the interpretation of the data. (Read Chapter 6 for an overview of LDX and other stimulants.)

It might sound like a conflict of interest for Shire to fund a study of their own medication, but this is the way research on new medications is performed in this country. Very few medication trials are sponsored by the government, universities, or another neutral party. Until a better system emerges, the veracity of the study data depends on the integrity of the researchers. Indeed, Shire took a hands-off approach to the project and in no way tried to influence me or the outcome of the study.

Off-Label Prescribing

Off-label prescribing refers to ordering a medication for a patient which has not been specifically designated for a disease or disorder based on recommendations from the Food and Drug Administration (FDA). The practice is common, and doctors often order medications off-label based on their experience and knowledge that these medications may help. Sometimes doctors discover that a medication works well for a condition, and then the FDA later approves it for that condition. For example, duloxetine (Cymbalta) was approved by the FDA in 2004 for depression, but it became apparent that certain types of back pain responded to duloxetine. Subsequent clinical studies verified this, and in 2010, this drug was approved for the treatment of musculoskeletal pain, osteo-arthritis, and low back pain.[1] Prior to this label update, all duloxetine prescriptions for back pain were off-label. One of the most commonly prescribed medication for insomnia, trazodone does not have an FDA indication. Lisinopril has an FDA indication for hypertension but is also commonly used off-label for coronary artery disease.[2]

This does not mean that every off-label use of a drug will be approved by the FDA. Early studies help develop the agenda for further research. Good ideas take root if they are rational and are proven by independent clinicians. New medical practices should be adopted after sober analysis; an FDA indication should only be granted after intense scrutiny.

In an era where doctors are moving away from using opioid medications, the search for safer agents to treat conditions involving chronic pain and fatigue need to be vigorously pursued. For the sake of our CFS patients, I am hopeful that over time, LDX (Vyvanse) will be subjected to multicenter, double-blind trials seeking to confirm or disavow the safety and efficacy of this new approach.

Notes

1. Katrina Woznicki, "FDA Approves Cymbalta for Chronic Musculoskeletal Pain," WedMD, November 5, 2010, https://www.webmd.com/pain-management/news/20101105/fda-approves-cymbalta-for-chronic-musculoskeletal-pain (accessed July 11, 2019).

2. Susan Ipaktchian, "14 Drugs Identified as Most Urgently Needing Study for Off-Label Use," Stanford University News Center, November 24, 2008, https://med.stanford.edu/news/all-news/2008/11/14-drugs-identified-as-most-urgently-needing-study-for-off-label-use-stanford-professor-says.html (accessed August 6, 2019).

Study Details

To enroll for the study, we reached out to both our existing clinical patients and the general public. We publicized the study through local newspaper and web advertising and benefited from referrals from two local hospitals. The recruitment efforts worked, and we received a flurry of phone calls of willing participants. The next phase was selecting the appropriate participants.

Our study was limited to adults diagnosed with CFS between 18 and 60 years old. To be eligible for the study, patients were screened for

CFS. As many people with CFS have other psychiatric conditions, we did not exclude potential subjects if they also had anxiety, depression, or ADHD. Many patients with CFS report difficulties in their ability to organize and in overall working memory, and we were especially interested to see if LDX helped these cognitive conditions. Subjects who did not have moderate-to-severe impairment at baseline were excluded from the study. Anyone with untreated hypertension, thyroid disease, or other medical problems for whom a stimulant would be a bad idea were excluded. No one who had previously taken LDX for any reason could participate.

The participants who qualified for our study ranged from ages 21 to 59. All of the subjects were female except for one. Early in the process, two groups were randomly assigned: one group to the active agent (LDX) and the other group to placebo. It turned out that 15 individuals joined the LDX group and 11 entered the placebo group. Unfortunately, four participants who had been preassigned to the placebo group did not enter the study because they ended up not qualifying. In retrospect, we should not have preassigned participants before they were randomized. However, although this was a technical mistake, I do not believe it changed the outcome of the study in a meaningful way.

The study was designed to last six weeks, and measurements on various scales were made at predetermined intervals. The LDX group was started at a dosage of 30 mg per day. If this dosage was tolerated, then after one week, it was increased to 50 mg per day. If that mid-range dosage was also well tolerated, then we administered the highest dosage of 70 mg per day. Equivalent modifications were made in the placebo group as well. The active drug and the placebo looked the same, so participants did not have a visual cue regarding whether they were receiving the LDX or the placebo.

At the beginning of a formal study, the protocol identifies one primary and several secondary outcome measures. The Behavior Rating Inventory of Executive Function-Adult (BRIEF-A) is an instrument that tests executive functioning (EF) skills, and it also nicely reflects changes over a short period. For this reason, it was a good instrument to assess the primary outcome measure we were looking for, which was cognitive changes in CFS. The secondary outcome measures were included to assess the levels of fatigue and pain in the subjects. Here we used the Fatigue Severity Scale (FSS), the McGill Pain Questionnaire (MPQ), and the Fibromyalgia Impact Questionnaire (FIQ). Other secondary outcome measures included the ADHD-Rating Scale (ADHD-RS) and the Hamilton Anxiety Rating Scale (HAM-A). Finally, we employed the Clinical

Global Impression-Improvement Scale (CGI-S) to assess changes in overall functioning. These rating scales were administered at the beginning and end of the trial. Safety is the paramount concern of every human trial; we assessed both blood pressure and pulse throughout the study.[1]

A Dive into Executive Functioning

CFS patients report that they have trouble with planning and organization. They also describe impaired concentration as well as difficulties starting and completing tasks and shifting to new tasks. Rapid mood swings can interfere with their daily functioning. This "emotional lability" represents the tendency to overreact to everyday stress or to experience heightened irritability. These functions contribute to EF, and these deficits are associated with the concept of brain fog, which is covered in Chapter 9.

Study Findings

The RCS showed that the group receiving LDX demonstrated significant improvement in executive skills compared to the group treated with placebo. The improvements in total EF as measured by the BRIEF-A in the LDX group were impressive; for example, at the end of the study, the placebo group improved 3.36 points, but the LDX group improved 21.38 points from their baseline score. This improvement is considered statistically significant, meaning that the change could not be considered accidental and was almost certainly associated with the use of LDX.

In looking at individual components of the BRIEF-A scale, some of the improvements were dramatic. For example, in the placebo group, the ability to plan and organize from the start of the study to the end improved by less than a point (0.64 points); however, the average score of the LDX group improved by 23 points. Furthermore, the working memory of the placebo group improved by 1.09 points. This improvement was minuscule compared to the memory improvement noted by the LDX group (21.46 points). Without exception, in this study, executive function scores significantly improved in the LDX group.

Considering Fatigue Changes

The unremitting exhaustion stemming from CFS concerns CFS patients as much as their cognitive complaints. To assess this symptom, we used the FSS. The FSS is a 9-item scale that assesses the impact fatigue has on the individual's motivation, exercise, and other physical and routine responsibilities. The FSS also quantifies self-image and the effect fatigue has on family relationships. Each item can be scored 1 to 7, with higher scores equating to more severe complaints.

As was seen with the EF scales, major improvements in fatigue were observed following the administration of LDX. Over the course of the trial, the baseline to endpoint improvement in fatigue was 5.08 points for the placebo group, but it was a hefty 20.92-point improvement for the LDX group. This level of improvement was robust and meaningful to the subjects with CFS.

Evaluating Pain in CFS

A subgroup, not all patients with CFS, complains of generalized pain. This is a low-level, chronic discomfort distinct from the sharp pain one might expect after surgery or a physical injury. Often the pain is musculoskeletal and takes the form of persistent achiness and tenderness. The pain might migrate throughout the body but is most often in the neck, jaw, and joints. Most characteristic of this type of pain is that doctors cannot seem to find an anatomical explanation. X-ray images or CT scans of the areas of concern do not reveal significant abnormalities. Sometimes the patient is told she has mild arthritis, inflammation, or a bit of bone degeneration, but the pain usually does not retreat with time and does not respond to anti-inflammatory medications.

The RCS used two scales to capture pain symptoms. The MPQ is a validated scale that takes about five minutes to complete. Subject responses, on a scale of 0–3, describe the presence and intensity of many different pain complaints. Among other descriptions, they can report throbbing, shooting, stabbing, exhausting, aching, or gnawing pain. Pain complaints can be summarized using adjectives such as, none, discomforting, horrible, or excruciating.

The second pain inventory used was the FIQ, which was developed at the Oregon Health and Science University in the 1990s and has since been revised. The FIQ surveys functional impact and allows the patient to gauge, in light of their discomfort, their ability to participate in daily activities, including shopping, preparing meals, and doing yard work. The questionnaire is very sensitive to change, so it is a useful instrument to use in short-term medication study. The FIQ was validated in fibromyalgia patients, but because a similar instrument did not exist for CFS, it was used as a secondary outcome measure in the RCS.

Once we analyzed the LDX study, it was clear that subjects taking the active agent experienced more pain relief than those on placebo. The mean MPQ went down 10.38 points for those treated with LDX compared to a mean decline of 2.45 points in the placebo group. The FIQ also detected a decrease in pain impact in the actively treated group's mean decline (20.90 points) vs. mean decline in the placebo group (8.83 points).

Anxiety Improvements

The product warning for every stimulant medication includes the potential for increased anxiety. For this reason, the RCS tracked the HAM-A throughout this LDX study. The 14-item scale is widely used in psychiatric medication trials, as it carefully tracks anxiety-related symptoms.

Two findings are notable here: First, the patient population recruited into the study met the criteria for CFS. It was interesting that when we started the study, both the LDX and placebo groups had rather high levels of anxiety. This reflects the extent to which generalized anxiety is characteristic of CFS. Second, over the course of this six-week study, the group treated with LDX had a mean decline in the HAS scores of 11.31 points compared to the placebo-treated group, who experienced a mean decline of 6.18 points. Not only did LDX not worsen anxiety, but the reverse was true. The RCS data showed a trend (not full statistical significance) of an improvement in their baseline high level of anxiety.

The final secondary outcome measure was the Clinical Global Improvement Scale-Severity of Illness (CGI-S). This scale allows the investigator to rate the severity of a subject's illness on a 7-point continuum. A score of 1 indicates "normal, not ill at all," a score of 4 means "moderately ill," and a score of 7 represents "among the most extremely ill patients."

At the beginning of the study, the mean CGI-S score was 5.1 for the LDX group and 5.4 for the placebo-treated group. At the end of the study, the group treated with LDX improved by 1.92 points compared to a mean decline of .92 points in the placebo group. This was a statistically significant decline and part of the larger trend showing decreased severity of symptoms in the LDX group.

Looking at Side Effects

Researchers refer to undesirable responses to a medication as adverse events, though most people use the term side effects. Because the RCS was double blind, neither the study team nor the study subjects knew who was assigned to the active treatment arm vs. the placebo arm. The protocol demanded that all subjects be asked at every visit how they were tolerating treatment. The most common side effects were headaches, dry mouth, and insomnia. The RCS found that 15 percent of the LDX subjects had headaches, compared to 8 percent of the subjects in the placebo group. In addition, about 8 percent of the LDX group experienced insomnia and dry mouth, whereas no one in the placebo group had these two complaints.[2] (I talk more about the insomnia side effect in Chapter 6.) It was noted that none of these side effects interfered with the subject's ability to stay in the study. No life-threatening adverse events occurred.

As mentioned above, the overall effect of LDX in this study showed anxiety reduction, but it is noteworthy that two of the LDX subjects discontinued the study because of increased anxiety. Both subjects improved rapidly once they stopped LDX. The message of the RCS regarding anxiety is that LDX can increase anxiety in select subjects but decreases this symptom in many others.

Safety: Blood Pressure and Pulse Changes

Many clinicians predict that a person's blood pressure and pulse would significantly rise while taking a stimulant drug, but interestingly, RCS found only a minor change in vital signs. As a reminder, blood pressure is measured in millimeters of mercury; a pressure reading of 118/70 means the systolic pressure (SBP) is 118 and the diastolic pressure (DBP) is 70.

In our study, the placebo group started with a mean SBP of 119.5, and it slightly increased to 121.3 by the end of the study. By chance, the LDX group had a baseline mean SBP of 124.10, but at the end of the study, it dropped to 119.75, a slight decrease.

The DBP of the placebo group was an average of 78.15 at the onset of the study, and it was 79.20 at the conclusion of the study, a nonmeaningful change. For the LDX group, the average DBP was 78.60 at the start of the study, and it slightly increased to 81.05 by the end of the study.

As for the pulse, the placebo group started out with an average pulse of 81.55 beats per minute, but it dropped to 77.55 by the end of the study. In contrast, the average pulse of the LDX group increased from 73.60 at the baseline to 81.05 by the end of the study. Thus, the actively treated CFS group did have an average increase in pulse rate; the clinical significance of this change is unknown. This finding is consistent with other LDX studies and is reassuring news to prescribers and patients, defeating the contention that stimulant medications are uniformly associated with deleterious changes to vital signs.

Limitations of the RCS Study

The RCS is one of several studies that have found that stimulants improve the plight of patients with CFS. Similar to its predecessors, the RCS has some inherent limitations. It was conducted at a single site; the ideal data should be gathered at multiple independent centers. The number of subjects studied was small, and some technical mistakes regarding randomization were eventually recognized. As a result, more participants received active agent than placebo. Although women are more likely to have CFS than men, the RCS had a disproportionate number of women. Finally, RCBM is an established ADHD center, and it is possible that this introduced a selection bias, resulting in a higher number of ADHD patients recruited into the CFS study.

The Way Forward

Despite these concerns, the positive findings of the RCS open the doors of imagination. From the study, we glean that global CFS symptoms respond favorably to LDX. There are four specific findings: Compared to placebo, LDX improved cognitive deficits in subjects with CFS. CFS subjects treated with LDX reported less fatigue. Most surprising was the noted decline in the physical pain experience by the CFS subjects. Finally, subjects with CFS treated with LDX reported less generalized anxiety.

The RCS forces a rethinking of the properties and proper uses of stimulant medication. Most fundamentally, the RCS reveals that LDX provided relief to subjects with CFS who were experiencing cognitive deficits. This is an important finding; very few medications available in the marketplace sharpen cognitive skills. As many individuals with CFS are diagnosed with other cognitive complaints ranging from brain fog to post-concussive syndrome to early dementia (discussed further in Chapter 9), this finding has potentially extensive implications.

In the RCS, LDX-treated subjects with CFS experienced improvement in the core symptom of fatigue. This might be the most predictable finding—it is well-known that stimulants augment energy. Earlier studies (to be described in Chapter 6) have reported similar findings with CFS.

Taken together, these studies offer a data-confirmed finding that LDX, and probably other molecules similar to LDX, have strong anti-fatigue properties. I assert that the symptom of fatigue is highly prevalent, quite debilitating, and underappreciated as a source of human distress. Often, fatigue patients are misdiagnosed as having anxiety or depression and as a result are treated with inappropriate medications. In the future, I hope the diagnosis of CFS is considered more routinely. Medications such as LDX should occupy a prominent role as a treatment option for these patients.

An understanding of the way LDX helps ADHD patients may explain why the medication worked to decrease pain scores. In ADHD patients, LDX enhances concentration by decreasing distractibility. A classic example is that with treatment, ADHD patients are better able to stay focused on tasks that require sustained attention, such as reading. Treated patients will often report that they no longer need to reread a simple paragraph, and they are less distracted while performing mundane tasks such as unloading the dishwasher. The same model applies to pain in the distinctively different CFS patient. As LDX increases attentional focus and decreases distractibility, CFS patients are better able to filter out irritating muscle and joint pain. I believe it is this mechanism, played out in the cortical dopamine circuits, that accounts for the reduction in the FIQ and MPI scales. In this era, when American medicine is moving away from long-standing opioid use, LDX might emerge as an alternative for chronic pain relief.

The RCS also documents a reduction in overall anxiety. This contradicts the general belief that stimulants increase generalized anxiety, but it is consistent with what many LDX-treated patients have described to me over the years. The biochemical mechanism probably involves LDX effects on the basal ganglia and the prefrontal cortex via dopaminergic properties, but this model will need further refinement. For now, I can say confidently that treated patients report they can focus more easily and are less distracted by worrisome thoughts. For this reason, they feel less anxious and overwhelmed.

Considering the Case of Abby

Abby is 56 years old and has been married to her husband, Logan, for 25 years. She was referred to my office for ongoing treatment of anxiety and depression. Abby related that since the onset of menopause six years earlier, she felt drained all the time, as if her "mind was somehow trapped in mud." Abby felt achy and bloated much of the time. She slept poorly at night and often felt restless during the day. Of concern to Logan was that Abby was increasingly unreliable; she was late for appointments, forgot to pay bills, and got stranded on the interstate after failing to fill the car with gas.

A paralegal, Abby had received several warning notices about her declining performance, and she was apprehensive that she would soon be fired from her job. Fueling her despair was Abby's persistent worry that her symptoms stemmed from an undiagnosed medical condition or even a latent cancer. Her trusted family doctor examined her carefully and referred her to specialists. Abby's gynecologic checkups and mammograms were normal, as was a colonoscopy. Her blood tests revealed a normal thyroid level and complete blood count. After an extensive workup, Abby's doctor told her, "You have no clear medical illness and do not show evidence of cancer. I cannot find an explanation for your fatigue."

Abby started to cry when she learned of her nondiagnosis; she had desperately wanted to find an explanation. Sensing that Abby was still in distress, her doctor referred her for psychiatric evaluation, having little else to offer.

Abby greeted me with the following: "My doctor thinks I am crazy, so she sent me to you. You will probably agree. I don't think anyone knows what wrong with me. Is there any hope for me at all?" I listened and then carefully documented Abby's history.

- Age 16: Diagnosed with mild depression and prescribed with the antidepressant desipramine, which she recalled helped her. Treatment ended about a year later, uneventfully.
- Age 20: Left college after her third semester. Was placed on academic leave and told she had ADD and possibly a learning disorder. No treatment was pursued.
- Age 25: Broke her leg while ice skating and was grounded from active sports for several months. She put on weight during the injury and has gained an average of a pound per year since then.
- Age 32: Now with two small children, Abby became a full-time homemaker. Her weight escalated during her pregnancies, and she struggled to maintain a basic exercise schedule.
- Age 49: Her mother died, and her primary care doctor prescribed a three-month course of fluoxetine (Prozac) during her grieving stage. Abby did not request refills after the prescription ended.
- Age 50: Began experiencing lethargy, lack of initiative, and an overall lassitude. Failed trials of the antidepressant Lexapro and Effexor resulted in referral to my clinic.

After reviewing her comprehensive medical workup and psychological testing, I diagnosed Abby with CFS. I explained that her history was consistent with CFS and encouraged her to try a small dose of Vyvanse. Abby was ambivalent about my diagnosis and expressed fear that she might develop a dependency on the medication. I reassured her that the risks were minimal, and she consented to proceed.

Within about a week of treatment with Vyvanse, Abby called my office to ask if the medication was also an antidepressant. Told it was not, she seemed surprised, because her long-standing feelings of depression and fatigue were essentially gone. Her performance improved at work, and her supervisor observed that Abby must have gotten her pep back, because she was doing so much better. Abby began going out with old friends she had not seen for years, to their mutual pleasure. She no longer needed to nap during the day, and her neck pain diminished to the extent that she was not taking ibuprofen. Instead of needing massages, she was working out in the gym three days per week and had lost 12 pounds. Three months into treatment, Logan came into our office to thank us for "giving me my wife back." He said he didn't know what happened to her or why it had happened, but that Abby was her old self again, and he was extremely relieved and happy.

This chapter concentrated on the RCS and the use of LDX in treating patients with CFS. The next chapter will explore all the stimulants that may be helpful to individuals with CFS, both long-acting and short-acting drugs. In addition, I will also discuss modafinil, a drug that promotes wakefulness and that been found helpful with chronic fatigue.

Notes

1. Joel L. Young, "Use of Lisdexamfetamine Dimesylate in Treatment of Executive Functioning Deficits and Chronic Fatigue Syndrome: A Double Blind, Placebo-Controlled Study," *Psychiatry Research* 207 (2013): 127–133.

2. Ibid.

CHAPTER 6

Understanding Stimulants and Their Role in Chronic Fatigue Syndrome

*J*ulie is a 36-year-old mother of two with a long history of seeking mental health treatment. She was a restless child prone to temper tantrums, and in fifth grade, she was too anxious to go to school for two months and refused to leave her mother's side. "I always felt overwhelmed and could not focus on learning," she explained. In middle school, Julie started to gain weight and became depressed. She attempted suicide at age 17, after which she sought counseling and medications.

Julie was accepted at a state university but had a disastrous first semester away from home. "My grades were terrible, and I didn't know what to do with my freedom," she recalled. "I drank too much and slept with too many guys. On one hand I had really bad self-esteem, and on the other hand, I discovered I had a lot of power over people, which I had never known I had before. I was so confused."

Julie ultimately completed her bachelor's degree, but it took almost six years. Afterward, she had no trouble finding a job. "I interviewed well and would always get hired but became bored easily and did not perform well on the job." Over the next few years, Julie went through nearly a dozen jobs. With her parents' guidance, she tried to get out of her self-defeating rut. She started a master's program but dropped out after a semester. She moved from Detroit to Chicago, immediately floundered, and had to move home within the year. Julie met her husband around this time; he was a recovering alcoholic who struggled with mood swings. They had two young children in three years.

After the birth of her first child, Julie gained 50 pounds, and after her second pregnancy, she was 80 pounds heavier than when she graduated high school. "I always had a problem relationship with food. It got worse when I was home with my children and started to binge-eat at night after the house settled down. I ate thousands of calories at a time, three or four times a week, and couldn't stop. I felt nothing but shame."

Julie also noticed that her fatigue intensified, and she spent every free moment in bed. "My husband and I essentially became roommates. He appreciated I was taking care of the kids, and I was content he was keeping us afloat." Eventually their strained marriage broke, and Julie and her husband divorced. "When I went back to work, I realized I was too fatigued to accomplish anything. It was just like after college when I went through so many jobs. My eating was out of control, and my family demanded I get help." Julie was relieved when the psychiatrist diagnosed her with binge-eating disorder (BED). She was placed on Vyvanse, a medication approved for this condition, and within the week, the frequency of her binge episodes decreased dramatically. "I also realized that I had had a lot more energy on the medication; I started to do better at work and was more effective with my kids," she said.

When Julie came to our clinic, she was panicked. "My insurance does not cover Vyvanse. This medicine has helped me with my chronic fatigue and binge eating, and I am doing better than ever." Our clinic drafted an appeal letter to Julie's insurance company, and after several exchanges, the company finally agreed to pay for the brand medication.

This chapter is about stimulants, including amphetamines, methylphenidate, and "wakefulness" drugs such as modafinil, that may help people with CFS. Keep in mind that the FDA has approved Vyvanse for ADHD and separately for BED. However, as of this writing, no medication has been approved for CFS. The RCS (Chapter 5) demonstrates that patients with CFS responded well to Vyvanse across a number of symptom domains. Unfortunately, Vyvanse is not available to everyone nor effective for everyone. Consequently, other medications that are stimulants or that are from a similar class should be considered. This chapter outlines stimulant medications that have been approved by the FDA to treat ADHD, BED, and some sleep disorders, and they may prove useful for CFS, as we found they did in our study described in Chapter 5.

There are three primary categories of prescribed stimulants: amphetamines, methylphenidate medications (which includes Ritalin and related medications),[1] and several different wakefulness-promoting drugs. Medications in this last category are non-amphetamine-like stimulant medications, the prototype being modafinil (Provigil). Throughout this chapter, I focus on medications that are good candidates for further research in the treatment of CFS. Note that physicians may prescribe medications off-label, which means not for their specific approved purpose.

At the onset, it important for readers to distinguish these safe and carefully studied medications from illegal stimulants such as cocaine or illegally manufactured methamphetamine. Cocaine and methamphetamine are dangerous, life-destroying drugs; they catapult the brain into a fevered and unhealthy state of euphoria and create an intense craving for more and more of the offending substance. Cocaine and methamphetamine play no role in therapeutic medicine and are rightly considered drugs of abuse.

Legal stimulant medications do not flood the brain; rather, they are taken up gradually into the central nervous system and do not cause euphoria. The chapter outlines prescribed stimulant medications and contrasts their lower risk for abuse and misuse compared to street stimulants and other drugs such as opioids and sedatives.

Considering Amphetamines

Amphetamines have been available to consumers for many years. In World War II, soldiers were given amphetamines such as Benzedrine to help them stay awake in combat conditions.[2] After the war, the drugs were prescribed for a surprising number of medical conditions, including the following:

- Alcoholism
- Allergies
- Asthma
- Menstrual problems
- Morphine addition
- Schizophrenia
- Seasickness[3]

It is no longer accepted that stimulants are effective for any of these conditions, but in the postwar era, it emerged that amphetamines were effective for children with hyperactivity. This category of medications is still used today, primarily to treat impaired concentration and focus in children, adolescents, and adults with ADHD. A few of the stimulant medications are used to treat narcolepsy; and, as mentioned, LDX (Vyvanse) is approved for BED.

An Accidental Discovery: Amphetamine Improved Behavior in Hyperactive Children

Charles Bradley was the first psychiatrist to publish research about the use of amphetamines with children. In 1937, Dr. Bradley was the director of the Emma Pendleton Bradley Home, a youth facility in Providence, Rhode Island. Upon admission to the hospital, many of the young patients were given a routine spinal tap, and this procedure led to persistent headaches. Desperate to find a solution for these headaches, Bradley tested many different medications but found the most interesting results when he administered the amphetamine Benzedrine.

We do not know if the children's headaches remitted with the amphetamine, but Bradley discovered that his patients' behavior and academic performance improved markedly subsequent to receiving the drug. When Bradley took the children off the Benzedrine, their behavior quickly reverted to previous low-functioning levels.[1] Until that time, it had been held that brain damage was the reason for severe hyperactive behavior. Later generations of physicians were dubious about the brain damage theory, and in 1972, physician Virginia Douglas at McGill University coined the phrase "attention deficit disorder," which is now called attention deficit/hyperactivity disorder (ADHD).[2] Although the debates about the causes and treatments of ADHD rage on, no one disputes that Bradley stumbled on one of the most important findings of 20th century psychiatry.

Notes

1. Christine Adamec, *Understanding Drugs: Amphetamines & Methamphetamine.* New York: Chelsea House, 2011.

2. Ibid.

Amphetamines May Improve Symptoms of Chronic Fatigue Syndrome

Treatments for CFS remain elusive, likely because most doctors cannot agree on the underlying cause. The current trend in chronic fatigue research is to explore the relationship between fatigue and inflammation. Much energy is being focused on imaging the brains of individuals with CFS and finding precise methods to measure inflammatory changes in the brain. Very little current work is being conducted on therapeutics and few treatment ideas for CFS are emerging on the horizon.

I organized a small but carefully executed clinical trial using the medication, Vyvanse. The details of the study are outlined in Chapter 5. The salient findings were positive: Vyvanse decreased fatigue and chronic pain and was also useful in lowering generalized anxiety.

Although the study revolved around Vyvanse, I believe that other stimulant medications also may be helpful. I want to emphasize that to date the FDA has not approved stimulants to treat CFS. It is my hope, however, that larger-scale studies will soon be undertaken to validate the use of stimulants in treating CFS.

Benefits and Risks of Amphetamines

When amphetamines are taken to relieve ADHD, many studies have shown the benefits of these drugs in helping individuals perform more effectively in their personal, work, and family arenas. Of course, as with many centrally acting medications, an amphetamine should be initially prescribed at a low dosage and then titrated upward, as needed.

Benefits of Amphetamines

In my study, Vyvanse was evaluated in patients with CFS. Relative to a placebo-treated group, the Vyvanse group demonstrated significant improvement in fatigue and pain. Interestingly, the participants taking Vyvanse also noticed a decline in their generalized anxiety. There is reason to believe that these benefits extend to other amphetamines. Vyvanse has the unique features of a prodrug, meaning that the drug is converted to an active medication once it transfers from the gut into the bloodstream. This prodrug mechanism allows for a long-acting effect. Other brand-name amphetamines offer different properties, such as a longer duration of action. Amphetamine medications are also available in less expensive generic formulations. Examples include generic versions of Adderall and Adderall XR, referred to as mixed amphetamine salts. (Table 6.1 lists the major amphetamines that are available as of this writing, as well as formulations of methylphenidate and other medications.)

Risks/Disadvantages of Amphetamines

There are some clear limitations regarding the use of amphetamines. Patients who have heart conditions, hypertension, heart failure, or rhythm disturbances should avoid these drugs. Amphetamine decreases appetite, and patients with low weight may not tolerate this side effect. Individuals with known hypersensitivity to amphetamines should pursue another treatment option. Of course, the medications are not always helpful; treatment it is a trial-and-error process, guided by the skill and experience of the physician.

Amphetamines are not indicated for people with hyperthyroidism or women who are pregnant. Women who are breastfeeding should avoid amphetamines as the drug can be present in their breast milk, and the impact on infants, while probably minimal, is unclear.

Common Side Effects of Amphetamines

Not everyone experiences side effects with amphetamines, but some effects commonly appear. Side effects typically decrease over time and include the following:

- Headache
- Weight loss
- Nosebleed
- Diarrhea
- Nausea
- Nervousness
- Dry mouth
- Changes in sex drive
- Painful urination
- Painful menstruation[4]

Severe side effects should be reported to the physician urgently and include:

- Paranoia
- Hallucinations
- Seizures
- Delusions (fixed false beliefs)
- Rash
- Mania
- Hives
- Unexplained wounds on the fingers and toes
- Swelling of the face, throat, tongue, eyes, or lips[5]

No Quantifiable Measurements with Psychiatric Medications

One disadvantage of any psychiatric drug—and this includes antidepressants, antianxiety medications, and stimulants—is that there are no easily quantifiable measurements to determine that yes, this is the proper medication or adequate dose of the medication. A finger stick will measure the blood sugar level in a patient with type 1 diabetes. The level is either normal, below normal, or above normal, and this information guides the physician to prescribe the correct dose of insulin. In contrast, psychiatrists prescribing behavioral medications must rely on patients to report whether and how their symptoms have changed. Fortunately, research studies employ standardized rating scales for fatigue, anxiety, and pain, and there are scales available for routine visits to the doctor that help inform decision making.

Dexamphetamine and Chronic Fatigue Syndrome

In a small study that predated our project, Australian researchers studied 20 patients with CFS. Ten subjects were assigned to a dexamphetamine treatment group, and the other half were given a placebo. The FSS was obtained at baseline and at the end of the study to compare differences that resulted from treatment. The medication group took one 5 mg tablet twice daily at 8:00 a.m. and again at 2:00 p.m. If there was no satisfactory therapeutic response after a week, the researchers increased the medication to 10 mg twice a day. After another week, if needed, the medication was increased to 15 mg. As it turned out, seven subjects stabilized at 10 mg twice daily (a total of 20 mg), and three of the subjects took three tablets or a dosage of 15 mg per day. The researchers found that nine of the medication subjects improved on the Fatigue Severity Scale, compared to four of the subjects taking the placebo. This was a statistically significant difference, indicating that the dexamphetamine did improve the fatigue of the study subjects.[6]

The researchers concluded:

> The use of dexamphetamine for chronic fatigue syndrome has a considerable degree of biological plausibility. The ability of dexamphetamine to antagonize the effects of sleep deprivation and increase alertness is among the best known of its actions, and symptoms similar, at least superficially, to those of sleep deprivation are very common in patients with chronic fatigue syndrome. In particular, difficulty sustaining concentration and slow recovery from exertion are among the most disabling symptoms of chronic fatigue syndrome, and the capacity of dexamphetamine to facilitate prolonged concentration and to allow renewed exertion without prolonged rest are prominent aspects of its action.[7]

In a subsequent publication, the lead author, Dr. Leslie Olson, expressed concern that short-acting amphetamines carry a double-edged sword.

They help cognitive symptoms, but as the dose wears off abruptly, the patient crashes hard, and the benefits are quickly overrun by this unpleasant side effect.[8]

Short-Acting or Long-Acting Amphetamines

Most experts agree that the duration of the effect of amphetamines affects the drug's safety and utility. It is important to understand the difference between short-acting and long-acting medications. In general, a short-acting amphetamine takes effect in about 30 minutes and may last up to four or five hours before its effects wane. In contrast, a long-acting drug lasts for 10 to 12 hours or longer, and intermediate-acting medications have a duration of effect somewhere between the two extremes. The amphetamine with the longest action is Mydayis, an amphetamine approved for ADHD in 2017. Mydayis lasts for up to 16 hours, and many doctors were concerned that it would cause insomnia. Clinical studies proved otherwise—only 2 percent of patients discontinued Mydayis because of poor sleep onset, and 94 percent with insomnia reported that their insomnia caused them only mild to moderate irritation. Most of the insomnia problems associated with this long-acting stimulant resolved over time.[9] (See Table 6.1 for more information.)

Considering the Various Types of Amphetamines

In this section, I provide information about the different types of amphetamines or amphetamine-like medications that are available in the United States. These drugs are listed in alphabetical order, as they also appear in Table 6.1. The amphetamine molecule can appear as *dextro*-amphetamine or its mirror image, *levo*-amphetamine. If the *d*-amphetamine and *l*-amphetamine are combined in equal proportions, it is called a *racemic* mixture. Many of the preparations on the market have varying proportions of *d* to *l* ratio, and this translates to slightly different clinical effects. Amphetamines ultimately affect the concentration of dopamine and norepinephrine, which are neurotransmitters jetting throughout the brain, particularly in the prefrontal region of the brain.

Adderall and Adderall XR

Adderall is the best-known amphetamine, introduced to market in the 1990s. This tablet consists of a ratio of three parts *d*-amphetamine to one part *l*-amphetamine. Adderall is a short-acting drug that is available in dosages of 5.0 mg, 7.5 mg, 10 mg, 12.5 mg, 15 mg, 20 mg, and 30 mg. The generic versions of Adderall are referred to as a mixed amphetamine salt.

Adderall XR is an extended-release formulation that was developed several years after Adderall. Adderall XR is a capsule with two different-sized beads. The smaller bead is absorbed within minutes after swallowing, and the larger bead is absorbed four hours later. Adderall XR exerts benefit for about seven or eight hours. It is available generically and comes in dosages of 5 mg, 10 mg, 15 mg, 20 mg, 25 mg, and 30 mg.

Adzenys XR-ODT

Adzenys XR-ODT is a long-acting drug manufactured by Neos Therapeutics, and it has the same *d* to *l* proportions as Adderall. This medication is distinctive in that it dissolves in the mouth and is appealing to people who do not like to swallow pills or capsules. Adzenys XR-ODT is orange-flavored and comes in dosages of 3.1 mg, 6.3 mg, 9.4 mg, 12.5 mg, 15.7 mg, and 18.8 mg.

Dexedrine and Dexedrine Extended-Release Spansules

Dexedrine is a short-acting amphetamine tablet consisting entirely of *d* amphetamine. Dexedrine extended-release spansules are an extended-release formulation that take an hour to become effective and last about six to eight hours. Dexedrine spansules are available in generic form in 5 mg, 10 mg, and 15 mg doses. All forms of dexedrine are generic medications.

Evekeo

Evekeo is a short-acting drug made by Arbor Pharmaceuticals. Evekeo is 50 percent *d*-amphetamine and 50 percent *l*-amphetamine. It is available in dosages of 5 mg, 10 mg, 15 mg, and 20 mg. Evekeo ODT is an orally dissolving preparation that is packaged in a convenient blister pack.

Mydayis

Mydayis is a long-acting medication designed to be taken in the morning. Mydayis was developed by Shire and is now owned by Takada. Mydayis is a triple-bead formulation with each bead consisting of the Adderall molecule. Like Adderall XR, the first bead releases immediately, followed by the second dose, which is released four hours later. Approximately eight hours after ingestion, the third bead is released, and this accounts for the 16-hour duration of action. Mydayis is available in capsule form in dosages of 12.5 mg, 25 mg, 37.5 mg, and 50 mg.

ProCentra

ProCentra is a sugar-free, bubble-gum-flavored fluid that is available from Independence Pharmaceuticals. This amphetamine is used primarily for children with ADHD but may be used by adults who are averse to swallowing capsules. As the liquid can be consumed quickly, the risk of diversion (illegally giving it to someone else) and overdose may be greater than in traditional capsule-based stimulants. Diverting amphetamines and other scheduled drugs to others is illegal.

Vyvanse

Vyvanse (LDX) was brought to market by Shire and is now manufactured by Takada. It is approved by the FDA as a treatment for both ADHD and BED. Vyvanse is a prodrug. This prodrug mechanism allows for a long-acting effect, and patients report benefit for 9 to 12 hours after taking the morning capsule. Vyvanse is available in dosages of 10 mg, 20 mg, 30 mg, 40 mg, 50 mg, 60 mg, and 70 mg. In contrast to Adderall and Mydayis, Vyvanse is not racemic and contains only *d*-amphetamine. The consumption of acidic substances such as fruit juices may decrease the effectiveness of the drug. In contrast, agents that decrease acid may increase its effectiveness.[10]

Zenzedi

Zenzedi, made by Arbor Pharmaceuticals, is a short-acting drug that is available in doses of 2.5 mg, 5.0 mg, 7.5, mg, 10 mg, 15 mg, 20 mg, and 30 mg. Like Vyvanse, Zenzedi is purely *d*-amphetamine.

Amphetamines and Methylphenidate May Raise Blood Pressure Only Slightly

Because amphetamines and amphetamine-like medications are stimulants, they may increase blood pressure somewhat, although usually not to the level of hypertension. Hypertension is defined as a blood pressure with a systolic blood pressure of 130–139 mm HG or a diastolic pressure of greater than 80.[1] For example, a person who has a blood pressure of 135/80 has high blood pressure, whereas a person whose blood pressure if 115/70 has normal blood pressure.

In large studies of stimulants in adult populations the typical increase in blood pressure was 2 to 4 mg of mm Hg. The average pulse elevations were four to six beats per minute.[2] Each physician will have to determine if their patient can tolerate these modest changes. It is best to measure blood pressure and pulse before a patient starts taking stimulants and then again, a month later, to ensure that these vital signs are within the normal range.

Individuals already diagnosed with hypertension are not good candidates for stimulant medications.

Notes

1. American College of Cardiology, "2017 Guideline for the Prevention, Detection, Evaluation, and Management of High Blood Pressure in Adults," *Journal of the American College of Cardiology* (September 2017), https://www.acc.org/~/media/Non-Clinical/Files-PDFs-Excel-MS-Word-etc/Guidelines/2017/Guidelines_Made_Simple_2017_HBP.pdf (accessed August 22, 2019).

2. Food and Drug Administration, "Vyvanse™ (lisdexamfetamine dinmesylate)," February 2007, https://www.accessdata.fda.gov/drugsatfda_docs/label/2007/021977lbl.pdf (accessed September 9, 2019).

Considering Methylphenidate Medications

Methylphenidate is the other stimulant that has been used for decades to treat children, adolescents, and adults with ADHD. It has also been used in adults with certain sleep disorders. Like amphetamine, methylphenidate affects the concentration of dopamine and norepinephrine in the brain, but its mechanism of action is less complex. Methylphenidate formulations are available in short-acting and long-acting formulations. (See Table 6.1.)

Benefits and Risks of Methylphenidate and Related Medications

The benefits and risks of methylphenidate medications essentially parallel the properties of prescribed amphetamines. When they work well, these drugs enhance concentration and focus and are effective at combating the hallmark symptom of CFS. In general, methylphenidate is less activating than amphetamine, and the class of methylphenidates may be less obvious candidates for formal study in CFS. There are numerous reports of misuse and abuse of methylphenidate, and clinicians should prescribe this medication with this risk in mind.

Methylphenidate and CFS

In a study of 60 patients with CFS, Blockmans and colleagues[11] found significantly decreased fatigue scores with methylphenidate. In this study, methylphenidate was given twice a day at a dose of 10 mg each (20 mg per day) over a one-year period. Subjects were randomly assigned to either the medication group (the study group) or the placebo group (the control group). The research team found that concentration problem levels in the medication group decreased significantly when compared to the control group.

The researchers were surprised to find that muscle pain also decreased in the methylphenidate group. They wrote, "An unexpected finding of our study was that muscle pain was scored significantly lower with methylphenidate than at baseline or with placebo." In addition, the researchers noted that methylphenidate was not associated with increased sleep disturbances.[12]

Looking at Types of Methylphenidate Related Drugs

There are multiple different brands and formulations of methylphenidate, and I discuss them next.

Adhansia XR

Adhansia-XR is produced by Purdue Pharma and is available in dosages of 25 mg, 35 mg, 45 mg, 55 mg, 70 mg, and 85 mg. It is a long-acting drug taken once daily in the morning.

Aptensio XR

This drug, manufactured by Rhodes Pharmaceutical, is a long-acting capsule that is taken once daily in the morning. The following dosages are available: 10 mg, 15 mg, 20 mg, 30 mg, 40 mg, 50 mg, and 60 mg.

Concerta

This is a long-acting drug taken that is slowly release through an OROS osmotic technology. Concerta was the first long-acting methylphenidate and was brought to market by the ALZA Corporation and marketed by McNeil. Concerta is taken once daily in the morning and is available in the following strengths: 18 mg, 27 mg, 36 mg, and 54 mg.

Cotempla XR-ODT

Neos Therapeutics manufactures Cotempla XR-ODT, a rapidly dissolving form of methylphenidate. This long-acting medication is taken once in the morning and is available in the following dosages: 8.6 mg, 17.3 mg, and 25.9 mg.

Focalin/Dexmethylphenidate HCl Extended Release

Teva manufactures the generic form of what was formerly called Focalin. Dexmethylphenidate is the *d* isomer of methylphenidate, and it has slightly different clinical properties than the racemic mixture. Patients generally have a preference between the two different formulations and can decide after they try each separately. Short and long durations are available. The extended release version is taken once per day and is available in the following capsule dosages: 5 mg, 15, mg, 30 mg, and 40 mg.

Jornay PM

This long-acting methylphenidate drug is administered in the evening because its onset of action is delayed for 10 to 12 hours after ingestion. This novel engineering, approved by the FDA in 2018, was developed by Ironshore Pharmaceuticals. Jornay PM comes in capsules with multiple strengths ranging from 20 mg to 100 mg. Jornay PM is taken at 8:00 p.m. and becomes active upon awakening in the morning. Prior to the availability of Jornay PM, patients had to awaken, take their stimulant medication, and wait 30 to 60 minutes for the medication to take effect. This delayed-release technology is particularly helpful for patients who have trouble transitioning from sleep to wakefulness in the morning and benefit from the medication being present at therapeutic levels upon awakening.

Metadate CD

Metadate CD, manufactured by UCB Inc., is a long-acting capsule and consequently is taken once daily in the morning, usually before breakfast. It is also available as a generic drug manufactured by Teva. The capsules last about six hours and are available in the following dosages: 10 mg, 20 mg, 30 mg, 40 mg, 50 mg, and 60 mg.

Methylin and Methylin ER

Methylin comes in the form of chewable tablets, regular tablets, and a liquid solution. The extended-release tablets are available in a 20-mg dosage, and is a generic drug. The grape-flavored chewable tablets come in the following dosages: 2.5 mg, 5 mg, and 10 mg. These chewable tablets are short-acting. The chewable tablets are made by Shiongi Inc., which also makes the liquid form of the drug.

Quillichew ER/Quillivant XR

Quillichew ER is a chewable cherry tablet that is long-acting. It comes in dosages of 5 mg, 10 mg, and 15 mg and is related chemically to Quillivant, a long-acting liquid suspension. Both medications were brought to market by Pfizer and were designed for younger children who have trouble swallowing tablets or capsules. Pfizer has since exited the ADHD market and sold the medications to a smaller company. These medications are now owned by Tris Pharma.

Ritalin LA

Ritalin LA was made by Novartis Pharmaceuticals Corporation as a long-acting capsule. Teva now produces a generic form of Ritalin LA in capsules that are 10 mg, 20 mg, 30 mg, and 40 mg. Ritalin LA is a dual-bead capsule where 50 percent is released immediately and then 50 percent is released four hours after the capsule is swallowed. The medication has a similar duration of action to Concerta of about nine hours, but compared to Concerta, it achieves greater effectiveness early in the day.

Daytrana

Daytrana is the only transdermal methylphenidate on the market. It is manufactured by Noven. Daytrana is applied to the upper buttock in the morning and removed later in the day. The manufacturer suggests a nine-hour wear time, after which the patch can be removed. The clinical effects dissipate over the next hour, ensuring no interference at bedtime. Adolescents and adults who initiate sleep later at night wear the patch for longer periods to obtain performance later into the evening. When Daytrana was initially introduced, there were some problems with adherence to the skin. This has been largely resolved, but because the patch can cause local irritation, it is suggested that the application site be alternated each day.

Possible Side Effects of Methylphenidate and Derivatives

As with amphetamines and related drugs, methylphenidate and derivative medications may also cause some side effects. Some of these side effects may include the following:

- Headache
- Decreased appetite
- Dry mouth
- Stomach cramps
- Weight loss
- Grinding of the teeth (bruxism)
- Nervousness

- Decreased sexual desire
- Heavy perspiration
- Muscle tightness

If any of the following symptoms or signs occur, the patient should see a physician right away or seek emergency medical help:

- Seizures
- Frequent painful erections or an erection that lasts longer than four hours
- Pain, numbness, or sensitivity to temperature in the fingers and toes
- Paranoia
- Agitation
- Changes in vision or blurred vision
- Blistering or peeling skin
- Hives
- Chest pain
- Shortness of breath
- Hallucinations
- Delusions

Stimulants and Drug Schedules

Prescribed stimulants are also scheduled drugs, which means that they are controlled by the Drug Enforcement Administration (DEA). There are five schedules, ranging from I to V. Schedule I drugs are all illegal and include such drugs as heroin and illegally manufactured methamphetamine. Marijuana is also a Schedule I drug under the DEA's schedules, although at least half the states in the United States have approved "medical marijuana," and some states allow the recreational use of marijuana among adults ages 21 years and older.

Schedule II drugs are medications that the DEA has determined have a high risk of abuse, and nearly all opioids (except for cough syrup with codeine) lie within Schedule II. Other drugs that are scheduled include sedatives such as barbiturates, sleep medications, and other medications that have some level of risk associated with them. In addition, most stimulants also lie within Schedule II, although wakefulness drugs like modafinil lie within Schedule IV. Because of this scheduling, some people are reticent to take stimulants because they fear that they might get addicted. The reality is that most people who encounter drug dependency are addicted to illegal drugs or to prescribed opioids. Prescribed stimulants rarely cause clinical dependency. To be sure, street stimulants such as cocaine or methamphetamine are trafficked and abused, but these illegal drugs were never intended for any medicinal value.

Numerous clinical studies explore the distinction of abuse potential between opiates and stimulant medications. For example, in 2015, Cassidy and her colleagues surveyed 10,000 people ages 18–49 years on their nonmedical use of scheduled stimulant drugs, including Adderall, Adderall XR, Concerta, Ritalin, and Vyvanse. The researchers also considered the lifetime nonmedical use of pain medications, sedatives/tranquilizers, and sleep medications. They found that the lifetime nonmedical misuse or diversion of any of these scheduled prescription drugs was 35 percent, meaning that more than a third of the respondents admitted to these behaviors.[13] This sounds rather disturbing, but continue reading.

These researchers discovered that the most commonly abused drugs were pain medications (25%), followed by sedatives/tranquilizers (16%), sleep medications (10%), and, last, prescription stimulants (8%). In addition, they found that those individuals who were the most likely to misuse prescribed stimulants were ages 18–25.[14] Of note, many of the young people misusing the stimulants had symptoms that were consistent with attention deficit hyperactivity disorder (ADHD) diagnosis, and thus, it is likely that at least some of these individuals were self-medicating to improve their symptoms, rather than trying to obtain a mind-altering high. In fact, other researchers who have studied college students who misuse prescribed stimulants (the demographic group that is the most likely to misuse these drugs), the primary goal was to improve their school performance and grade point average. They might be surprised to learn that misusing the medication did not improve their grades.[15]

A 2005 study of 4,000 respondents ages 18 to 49 evaluated the non-medical use of Ritalin, Dexedrine Adderall, Adderall XR, and Concerta. The past-year prevalence of these "ADHD stimulants" was 4.3 percent among individuals ages 18 to 25 years and 1.3 percent among those ages 26 to 49 years. The most common type of misuse was giving the prescribed drug to friends and family members.[16]

As most people with CFS are typically older than age 25, the risk for misuse appears minimal.

Wakefulness-Promoting Drugs

Modafinil (Provigil) is one of several wakefulness-promoting drugs used to treat CFS. Modafinil, a non-amphetamine-like drug, is indicated for narcolepsy, a disorder in which a person has little control over falling asleep. Modafinil is also approved for patients with excessive sleepiness associated with sleep apnea and shift work sleep disorder (SWSD) a condition characterized by insomnia and excessive sleepiness affecting people who have inconsistent sleep schedules. Nurses and truck drivers notoriously suffer from SWSD, and the medication allows these shift workers to stay awake when needed until they transition to a new sleep/wake cycle.

In addition to modafinil, other wakefulness-promoting drugs include armodafinil (Nuvigil) and Sunosi (solriamfetol). Unfortunately, data is limited as of this writing, and carefully controlled studies have not been conducted with nonstimulants in CFS patients. My clinical experience is that they are effective in CFS and need to be systematically compared to long-acting stimulants.

Fatigued, Sleepy, and Depressed Patients Improved with Modafinil

In a study published in 2006, it was noted that some depressed patients treated with fluoxetine (Prozac), an antidepressant, continued to be sleepy and fatigued. In the six-week study, 21 patients were supplemented with 100 mg to 200 mg of modafinil in the morning. Each subject was evaluated with the Fatigue Severity Scale, the Epworth Sleepiness Scale, and the Hamilton Rating Scale for Depression at the onset of the study and at the second and sixth weeks of the study.

The results were positive; in this fluoxetine + modafinil study, all the patients improved in sleepiness and fatigue, and most of the subjects (76%) also improved in depression scores.[1] The take home message is clear. As many patients with chronic fatigue syndrome suffer from depression as well as sleepiness and fatigue, a trial of modafinil along with an antidepressant may be a consideration.

Note

1. Numan Konuk, et al., "Open-Label Study of Adjunct Modafinil for the Treatment of Patients with Fatigue, Sleepiness, and Major Depression Treated with Selective Serotonin Reuptake Inhibitors," *Advances in Therapy* 23, n. 4 (July/August 2006): 646–654.

Key Benefits and Risks of Wakefulness Drugs

Wakefulness drugs offer potential benefits to individuals with CFS. Wakefulness medications received Schedule IV classification from the DEA, meaning that this class of medication is less likely to be misused and diverted than Schedule II stimulant medications. The lower tiered scheduling offers other benefits as well. When a Schedule II drug is prescribed, the patient must obtain a new, separate prescription every month. In contrast, the medical provider can authorize multiple refills of Schedule IV medications. Another advantage is that doctors are less apprehensive about prescribing Schedule IV medications. Doctors are being scrutinized by state regulators about their use of controlled medication, and many states now issue a regular report card enumerating how many controlled substances a doctor wrote in the past three months. To avoid any appearance of impropriety, many providers are more comfortable prescribing nonstimulants, even if they do not feel these medications are safer or more effective than stimulant medications.

Wakefulness drugs may cause nausea, headache, anxiety, and difficulty with sleeping.

Modafinil and Chronic Fatigue Syndrome Recovery

Wakefulness medications have been studied to a very limited extent in CFS. In a case study of an afflicted 33-year-old man, Turkington and colleagues described Mr. C, who at age 19 complained to his physician of fatigue, poor sleep, and pain. He initially required complete bed rest, and over the next decade, he had periods of response and relapse. Eleven years later, Mr. C was in a wheelchair and could barely care for his basic needs. He was then treated with modafinil and clonazepam (an antianxiety medication) at a therapeutic dose. Upon receiving the medications, Mr. C reported significant improvement in his energy levels and noted sustained benefit from treatment. Dr. Turkington notes that the patient was sick for 13 years before he was finally diagnosed with CFS and treated for the condition.[17] As a practicing psychiatrist, I too have witnessed a significant number of patients who, like Mr. C, who have responded favorably to modafinil. More studies of wakefulness-promoting medication in the treatment of CFS would be welcome.

More on Modafinil

Modafinil (Provigil) is a "wakefulness" drug. It is owned by Cephalon Inc. and is available in tablets in dosages of 100 mg and 200 mg. Armodafinil is the generic form of modafinil, and it is also owned by Cephalon.

Sunosi

Jazz Pharmaceuticals owns Sunosi. This wakefulness drug, approved by the FDA in 2019, is available in tablet form in dosages of 37.5 mg, 75 mg, and 150 mg. It is a dual reuptake inhibitor drug, and it acts to increase the release of both dopamine and norepinephrine. It has not been formally studied in CFS.

Table 6.1 Medications That May Be Further Explored to Treat CFS

Name	Short-acting	Long-acting
Amphetamines and Amphetamine Derivatives, Brand Name (Generic Name)		
Adderall	√	
Adderall XR		√
Adzenys XR-ODT		√
Aptensio XR		√
Dexedrine	√	
Dexedrine spansules		√
Evekeo	√	
Mydayis		√
ProCentra (dextroamphetamine sulfate)	√	
Vyvanse (lisdexamfetamine)		√
Zenzedi (dextrianogetanube sulfate)	√	
Methylphenidate and Derivatives		
Adhansia XR		√
Concerta		√
Cotempla XR-ODT		√
Dexmethylphenidate HCl XR		√
Jornay PM		√
Metadate CD		√
Methylin	√	
Methylin ER		√
Quillichew ER		√
Quillivant XR		√
ProCentra	√	
Ritalin	√	
Ritalin LA		√
Wakefulness Medications		
Modafinil		√
Sunosi		√

This chapter has covered a number of medications that may help individuals with CFS, taking account both the risks and the benefits. In the next four chapters, I explore major features of CFS, including fatigue, chronic pain, brain fog, and sleep issues and offer suggestions on how to deal with these very troublesome symptoms.

Notes

1. N. G. Bradley and O'Brien, Angela, "Beyond ADHD and Narcolepsy: Psychostimulants in General Psychiatry," *Advances in Psychiatric Treatment* 15 (2009): 297–305.

2. Norman Ohler, *Blitzed: Drugs in Nazi Germany.* New York: Penguin Press, 2017.

3. Christine Adamec, *Understanding Drugs: Amphetamines & Methamphetamine.* New York: Chelsea House, 2011.

4. National Institutes of Health, "Amphetamine," *MedlinePlus*, April 15, 2019, https://medlineplus.gov/druginfo/meds/a616004.html (accessed August 23, 2019).

5. Ibid.

6. L.G. Olson, Ambrogetti, A., and Sutherland, D.C., "A Pilot Randomized Controlled Trial of Dexamphetamine in Patients with Chronic Fatigue Syndrome," *Psychosomatics* 44, n. 1 (January–February 2003): 38–43.

7. Ibid., page 42.

8. Leslie Olson, "The Difference: Nootropic vs. Amphetamines," *PharmaQuality*, May 15, 2017. https://pharmaquality.com/2017/05/15/the-difference-nootropic-vs-amphetamines/ (accessed September 6, 2019).

9. Jeffrey R. Strawn and Picard, Lara S. "Triple-Bead Mixed Amphetamine Salt for ADHD," *Current Psychiatry* 16, n. 8 (August 2017): 33–37.

10. Stephen M. Stahl, *Stahl's Essential Psychopharmacology Prescriber's Guide. Sixth Edition.* Cambridge, UK: Cambridge University Press, 2017.

11. Daniel Blockmans, et al., "Does Methylphenidate Reduce the Symptoms of Chronic Fatigue Syndrome?" *American Journal of Medicine* 119 (2006): 167e23–167e30.

12. Ibid.

13. Theresa Cassidy, et al., "Nonmedical Use and Diversion of ADHD Stimulants among U.S. Adults Ages 18–49: A National Internet Survey," *Journal of Attention Disorders* 19, n. 7 (2015): 630–640.

14. Ibid.

15. Amelia M. Arria, et al., "Do College Students Improve Their Grades by Using Prescription Stimulants Nonmedically?" *Addictive Behavior* 65 (February 2017): 245–249.

16. Scott P. Novak, et al., "The Nonmedical Use of Prescription ADHD Medications: Results from a National Panel," *Substance Abuse Treatment, Prevention, and Policy*, October 2007, https://substance abusepolicy.biomedcentral.com/track/pdf/10.1186/1747-597X-2-32 (accessed August 13, 2019).

17. Douglas Turkington, et al., "Recovery from Chronic Fatigue Syndrome with Modafinil," *Human Psychopharmacology Clinical and Experimental* 19 (2004): 63–64.

PART 3

Treating Chronic Fatigue Syndrome and Resolving Key Symptoms

In this part of four chapters, I cover the key problems of severe fatigue, chronic pain, brain fog, and sleep disorders, offering as much practical advice as possible. Be sure to read all of these chapters.

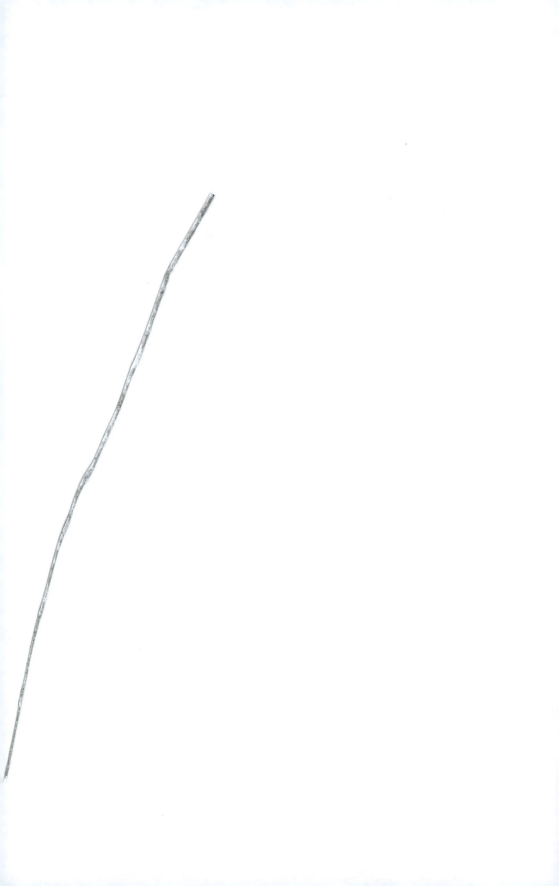

CHAPTER 7

Chronic Fatigue and Coping with Its Impact on Life

René

I manage my energy like a budget. I know that there is only so much of my energy to go around, and its first come, first serve. I make it to work every day, but barely. I try to get my work done: I know my job well, and no one is directly supervising me. I find it difficult to have enthusiasm for any new projects—I know this disappoints my boss, who is more of a cheerleader. There are times when I am sitting at my desk all day long, and if I am honest with myself, I get very little done. A bad day at work often becomes a bad day at home. When I feel so achy and spent, it's hard to come home and prepare dinner and get my kids ready for the next day.

René's Boss

René has worked for my family business for many years, and she's earned some independence. But I now have second thoughts about her role here. She barely does anything anymore. René does come to work, but she is pretty unapproachable. I find myself avoiding her; I just find someone else on the staff if I need help with a new project. For a while, I dealt with it. But now when I see her becoming impatient with a customer or not enforcing the new billing policy, I realize it's time for a change. I did not give her a raise last year.

René's Husband

It's a lot different than it used to be. She is so unhappy. Work saps her energy. René is exhausted when she comes home, and after an hour of the kids' homework, she goes right to bed. I am the only one who communicates with our kids' teachers. I don't think the teachers even know who she is. You would think it would be better on the weekends, but no. René sleeps in and does not want to do anything fun. I have just learned to plan things around her. She pretty much neglects me and my needs, and I am really angry—and it shows.

Living with CFS is challenging, as anyone who suffers from this medical problem can attest. In some cases, CFS forces harsh decisions, and it seems like every choice requires an automatic opportunity analysis. Do I really need to expend energy doing this? How can I not do that? Whom will I disappoint if I don't go there? Not only must the patient live with the physical symptoms, but she must also confront the fallout her behavior has on all those around her. CFS, of course, is a silent disability; most sufferers find that sympathy and understanding are very scarce resources.

This chapter considers the impact of CFS on the lifestyles of people who have the condition and discusses methods to overcome this fatigue. Some researchers have estimated the economic burden of CFS into hundreds of millions, perhaps even billions, of dollars. It's easiest to quantify the cost in terms of the high medical expenses, such as doctor visits and prescription drugs. Accounting for the individual's lost productivity is harder to measure; absenteeism constitutes a larger part of this cost, as does "presentism," which is a term that refers to being at work but accomplishing little while there. In turn, insurance companies and the federal government pay billions in payments to individuals disabled by CFS and the medical conditions closely linked to it, such as fibromyalgia, chronic pain syndromes, and treatment-resistant depression and anxiety. These are expenditures spread over the entire population, indirectly affecting health care costs, insurance premiums, and even taxes.

Imagine someone like René, operating in her own small sphere, both at home and at work. Then extend the ripple effect outward to all the other many people with CFS, and soon you can see that their plight has a major impact on their families and their workplaces. The impact does not have to be negative. The goal of this book is for readers to take better control over their CFS and their lives. The greater the independence the individual with CFS can attain, the lighter the burden of the disease is on herself and others.

The highest cost is to the patient with CFS and their family. CFS is insidious; quietly, over time, it sweeps up many victims. Living with CFS affects one's own sense of self and alters how the patient views work and relationships. In this chapter and throughout the book, I have used case studies and other interview techniques to paint this picture. The case studies revolve around patients I have cared for and known for years. I have made every effort to disguise them, to the extent that I doubt that anyone would recognize themselves, as I value their privacy and appreciate the chance to communicate their stories.

Interactions with Family Members

Sometimes interactions with specific family members are positive, but usually the reception is quite mixed. Many people with CFS were eager to describe how their families have dealt with their illness.

- My husband and daughter have been very supportive, and they recognize the early signs that I am overdoing things and often tell me to rest. Apparently, my stride changes, and my speech starts to slow down. They see this happening and know that it's time for me to take a break—and tell me so.
- My husband and children would walk over hot coals for me, but my sisters and my parents—they just don't get it, or they don't want to get it. I've given up trying to explain my illness to them.
- My husband and I work together, and he has always insisted I continue to work no matter how much I've wanted to quit. There have been times when I wanted to go home at lunchtime, and he insisted that I finish out the day and said I could nap when I get home.

Amber and Elliot: CFS in a Young Marriage

Amber was referred to me by the local hospital. On two consecutive Saturday afternoons, she presented to the emergency room late at night with chest pain. Both times she was convinced that her fast heart rate and labored breathing were signs of a heart attack. The ER staff did an extensive workup; they even arranged for Amber to see a cardiologist the next day. No heart disease was detected, and she felt some temporary reassurance. A week later, Amanda returned to the hospital with the same symptoms. Fortunately, the same doctor saw her during both of her visits, and they developed an easy trust. The doctor was not quick to diminish the sincerity of Amber's complaints; she was not offended by his honesty. When the doctor explained to Amber that she was having panic attacks rather than cardiac symptoms, she quietly agreed. They both thought it was a good idea for her to visit with a psychiatrist.

Two days later, I saw Amber in my office. She explained that she had completed her PhD several months earlier and recently been hired as an assistant professor at a local university. Now in her first semester of teaching, Amber was leading three freshman classes. "There is so much pressure on me. We have a new dean, the building I work in is under renovation, and my students don't respect me." She continued, "I have been through a lot. I have been a graduate student for the past ten years, and my husband and I anticipated that we would have more fun and freedom once I started this new job. It's actually worse than before."

Amber offered me more background. She was always an excellent student. In high school, she had played lacrosse and basketball and earned a scholarship to Johns Hopkins University. She played two years for their team and then lost interest once her recruiting coach left. In her junior year, she diverted all her energies to study. Amber was highly regimented, studying many hours during the school year and completing desirable summer internships. She was recruited to Harvard and contributed to several important research articles while there. On graduation day, Amber was honored by her faculty, and more than one professor remarked that "she did everything we asked of her." Throughout her education, Amber had one boyfriend, Elliot, and their relationship evolved without much drama. They were married several weeks after graduation in an elaborate wedding planned entirely by Amber's mother. Two weeks later, the couple moved to her new post as a junior faculty member at a top Midwestern university. Elliot found an engineering job at General Motors.

Since her senior year in college, Amber has reported high levels of anxiety and profound sensations of fatigue. Her father took her to many physicians in her late adolescence, and she was started on antidepressant medication. This medication quieted her panic attacks, but her lethargy continued. After a while, she stopped asking the doctors about her chronic fatigue. When I met her, Amber had been on a stable dose of the antidepressant sertraline (Zoloft) for six years.

I asked Amber if there was any significance to her coming to the ER on two consecutive Saturdays. "Maybe. During the week, I know exactly what to do. My classes start at eight a.m., and my last class is out at four p.m. On days that I don't teach, I have busy office hours. Faculty meetings and my research lab structure my other weekdays."

What about the weekends? "Bad time for me!" Amber responded. "I don't want to wake up on weekends because Elliot wants to get out and do things. I don't have the energy to make plans. When he asks me what we are doing or where we are going shopping, I shut down. I get irritable. I can't make myself socialize, and I just want to stay in bed. There was a small faculty party the other night, and I told them I was sick. I can't keep using the sick excuse with Elliot anymore. He is getting really bored and resentful. I am worried that he is losing faith, which is so sad because we worked so hard to get here, and it's a disaster."

I wondered whether the troubles encountered by this high-functioning woman were due to being far from home, starting a formidable job, or adjusting to a new marriage. I questioned Amber whether she may have married prematurely or was having second thoughts about taking her new job. She rejected each of these suggestions. "It's not the job, it's not the new city, it's not Elliot; it's my fatigue," Amber lamented. "I feel bad that I muster just enough energy to get through my week, and I have nothing left to give my husband." She added, "I love him, but I hate that I am disappointing him so much. I should be able to unpack and organize my stuff or go with him to the store to buy some new things. But I just can't find the energy to get it done." Amber reported that she makes every effort to appear upbeat for her students and colleagues. "I'm a perfectionist and a good actor, but I can't fake the same attitude at night and on weekends."

I spent some time talking to Elliot, too. He was angry and frustrated and not feeling charitable toward his new wife.

"I just don't know what's wrong with her. All she does is stay in bed. She seems to do okay at work, but when she is with me, we do nothing. I work with lots of talented people, and they all do things after work. I go home to Amber, and she is totally unavailable. She has no interest in sex. I have even gone to the casinos a few times just to have something to do. It's so bad, the blackjack dealers now recognize me." At the next appointment, Elliot announced that he planned to leave if things did not improve with Amber. "It's not a threat—that's not my style. It's just that I signed up for one person and was delivered another."

Amber's case is typical of a person with CFS. CFS can affect the young and old, high school dropouts and Ivy League graduates. It causes deep psychological burdens and distorts family relationships. With that understanding, this book is intended to cover the best ways of diagnosing CFS and differentiating it from other medical and psychiatric conditions. Effective treatments, including medications, counseling, and behavioral changes, are thoroughly discussed. The good news is that treatment ultimately did help Amber. Her relationship with Elliot greatly improved, and she began to thrive at work.

For People with CFS, Sustained Exercise Lowers the Pain Threshold and Increases Pain

There are those who believe that exercise is the key to nearly every problem, including chronic fatigue. Although some exercise may be beneficial, researchers have found that exercising as if one did not have chronic fatigue may be misguided. For example, in one small study of five subjects with CFS and five healthy subjects, researchers found that exercise *lowered* the pain threshold. This translated into more pain for the subjects with chronic fatigue earlier than it did for the healthy controls. For CFS patients, pain seem to be intensified by trying to exercise at the same level as people without the condition.

In this study the exercise comprised three five-minute periods of exercise on a treadmill, with increasing inclines of the treadmill at each stage. The CFS subjects were ages 28–49, and the control subjects were ages 30–54. Pain levels were evaluated by using pressure on the skin at the start of the exercise, after each exercise period, and 20 minutes after the final exercise. Exercise increased in the pain levels in the controls which means they could tolerate pain better, but the opposite effect occurred with the CFS subjects.[1] This small study concluded that if people with chronic fatigue syndrome exercise, they need to stop sooner than people without CFS. They should not try to "keep up" with their peers in terms of exercise.

Note

1. Alan Whiteside, Hansen, Stig, and Chaudhuri, Abhijit, "Exercise Lowers Pain Threshold in Chronic Fatigue Syndrome," *Pain 109* (2004): 497–499.

Relationships with Friends and Coworkers

Most of us spend a good deal of time at work, and relationships with coworkers can be both exhilarating and exasperating. Through our Facebook survey, we asked individuals with CFS to talk about the impact of their symptoms on their work life. Their experiences varied:

• No one has a clue as to how I really feel. I stopped trying to explain how I feel after a coworker told me that I did not get enough sleep and that was the only reason I was so tired and missed so much work.

- I pulled myself together to have lunch with a senior colleague with whom I had worked in the past. She had mentored me, and I felt comfortable telling I her about my CFS. She barely let me describe my condition before she blurted out that she had the same thing for a few weeks. She took some supplements she found on-line and insisted that all I needed to do was to take the mineral and I'd be fine. She made it sound so easy. If she had listened, I would have told her of the many medications, supplements, and other remedies I had used for my fatigue. It was then I realized how little she really understood me and the condition, and I was so annoyed that I changed the subject. I left lunch feeling even more alone.
- I have an understanding boss. She has known me for a year, and we talked about my chronic fatigue. Her sister has CFS, and she knew a lot about it. When my grandmother died, she noticed that I could not go to her funeral because I was unable to find the strength. A few people at work wonder if I am putting on an act, but most are supportive. My boss knows that I sincerely want to get the work done. She offered to let me work remotely, and I only come into the office two times a week. I miss the camaraderie of the office, but remote working has made me more effective. I am worried that my next boss won't allow this arrangement to continue.

Olivia and Work

Olivia became my patient in 2013, and my first meeting with her was not ideal. Thirty years my junior, she had no trouble expressing how disappointed she was that she could not find a female doctor, that she had to wait a few weeks to see me, and that the appointment started at 2:15 p.m., 15 minutes after it was scheduled. She was a professional manager, she explained, and punctuality was of utmost importance.

Olivia explained that she had just been transferred to the Detroit suburbs from Washington, D.C. There, she had worked as a restaurant manager for a growing upscale steakhouse, and because of her stellar performance, she was promoted to open a new location down the street from my office. Olivia was on an antidepressant medication and was only interested in finding a doctor to continue her care. She did not feel the need to reevaluate her diagnosis and elected to forgo our standard practice of diagnostic testing for new patients. "I'm fine. I just need someone to fill my Lexapro." This first interaction with Olivia was unsatisfying, but I acquiesced and refilled her antidepressant.

Olivia returned a month later. Still arrogant, she reported that things were not going well at the new restaurant. Several new hires had left abruptly, and she was doing the job of three people. "I am exhausted! I stay at work for eighteen-hour shifts just to get things done." She made an unexpected appointment two weeks later and told me that senior management in D.C. was sending her an assistant manager. "I am relieved that headquarters knows how hard this location is—once they get here, they will see what a mess I inherited."

Three weeks later, Olivia came to my office, this time in tears. "I was fired. They said I was doing terribly. All the cooks and wait staff said I was impossible to work for. Nobody supported me. I came all the way to this city, and I was let go. I don't know what to do."

With few options at this point, Olivia knew she had to do things differently. She sat for psychological testing and opened up in therapy. Although she initially presented in a secure, polished fashion, Olivia's testing revealed high levels of both depression and anxiety. She also reported having long-standing problems with concentration and distractibility. Her fatigue score was in the 90th percentile when compared to other women her age.

I sat down with Olivia and shared the results of the testing. "I think you have depression, ADHD, and chronic fatigue syndrome."

After a moment, she responded, "I don't disagree. When I was younger, I was treated for ADHD. When I started working in the restaurant business, I did not have insurance, so I could not get my ADHD medications filled. Everyone in the kitchen had cocaine, and after work, we partied every night. At my last job, my boyfriend was a dealer, and I used cocaine all the time. I think it made me awesome at work. I had so much energy that I looked like a superstar. I moved here to get away from the coke and my controlling boyfriend. Without it, I learned that I could not function, but I thought the feeling would pass. It didn't."

Olivia continued, "I became explosive to everyone around me. Even weeks after stopping the cocaine, I could not motivate myself to organize anything at the restaurant. All the people I hired quit after a few weeks. I was at work all the time, but I got nothing done. Since I was fired, I have been in my apartment sleeping all day for weeks. I feel so sad to realize that the success I had at my previous job was just cocaine driven."

Olivia agreed to treatment for her ADHD, and to her delight, her fatigue improved as well. She found a new job in a catering business. She met and married a family physician and decided to stay in the Detroit area. She now manages their busy practice and is responsible for its rapid growth. Seven years after I met Olivia, she remained on ADHD and antidepressant medications. Her craving for cocaine stopped once her ADHD and fatigue were addressed.

"I do so much better when I am on ADHD medication. During my pregnancy, I didn't take anything. I was exhausted and really could not work, but I knew it was for a short period. I can tolerate the discomfort when I know there is light ahead." Olivia decided not to breastfeed her second infant so she could return to medications immediately after delivery. "My son can thrive with formula, but I can't function without my medications. It is really important that I feel well so I can be at my best for him and for my job."

CFS Affects Self-Esteem

CFS directly interferes with self-esteem as a person's self-assessment. Self-value is eroded every time the person is unfairly accused of being lazy or seeking the fast track to disability. CFS involves more than feeling tired; it's a feeling that your body weighs a ton and you cannot move it. You need to move it, and you want to move it, but you just can't. CFS is not simply being overworked or stressed out. Rest or relaxation is not the magic elixir. People with CFS may know that the condition is not of their making, but they still blame themselves and assume that somehow, they are contributing to their own suffering.

Our Facebook survey inquired about self-concept. Some people passively accepted their condition, but most had little internal reserve to counteract the negative energy that CFS spawns. I have included a sampling of the various comments that respondents offered about how they feel about themselves in relation to their illness:

- For me, the hardest part about this problem is not knowing how I will feel from day to day, even if I have a few good days. It's not knowing how stress will affect me. Not knowing if the headaches will come back again, or the swollen neck glands, the trouble sleeping at night. Not knowing what is going to make me worse. Not knowing if I can talk to anyone about it. And not having anyone to relate to in my healing process. It's very lonely sometimes.
- People don't understand CFS; they think you get sick and then after a while, you get better—like when you get the flu. Or they think that if you're fatigued, then you should go to sleep, get some rest. But you can sleep for 10 or 12 hours with this thing, and then wake up, and you don't feel any better at all.
- I've mostly learned to live with it, but I cannot keep up with everything like I used to. I felt like a failure most of the time. I still do.

Men with CFS: Theo and JJ

CFS is not exclusively a women's malady; although women have a greater risk for CFS, men may also suffer. I met Theo and JJ many years ago and maintain a professional relationship with both. Although they do not know each other, I often wish I could introduce them. Both men have severe CFS, and both have received similar treatments. Their self-concepts could not be more different.

Theo and His CFS

Theo was referred to me by his primary care doctor. He was raised in Michigan but lives on a barrier island in South Carolina. He returns to Michigan regularly to visit his nieces and parents. Nearly 20 years ago, while in his 20s, Theo's partner died of an HIV complication. To his surprise, Theo inherited a large estate. Despite his wealth, he lives alone in a modest home and spends very little money on himself. He has not worked since his partner died and draws no disability income. Theo greets his Carolina neighbors warmly but makes little effort to engage anyone in his community. When he visits his family in Michigan, I see him to catch up and review his medications for CFS.

Very little happens between visits, and our visits took on a bleak routine. Several years ago, Theo started and then stopped renovating his increasingly dilapidated home. A hammer has not entered the doors in five years. His lives between the aluminum studs and seems not too concerned that another winter is coming. He does not act depressed and enthusiastically defends the effectiveness of Mydayis, the medication he takes for off-label for CFS. "Without my medicine, I would sleep all day and not even be motivated enough to pay my bills," he says.

Theo openly shared his self-disdain. "Why would I finish my house? It does not bother me, and I really don't invite anyone over. I have no interest in working. I am not a go-getter, and there is no boss who would put up with me."

"Theo," I asked, "You are living far from family—you must be lonely. Would you consider trying to find a new relationship?"

"No," he replied. "I have nothing really to add to anyone. I had a relationship so many years ago that now it doesn't even seem real to me."

Theo and I seem to have nearly the identical conversation every three months for the past decade. He tends to reject any new idea I have for him to improve his situation. I am confident that the medications he takes are on target; his fatigue is amplified if he does not take his medication, and on some level, he is benefiting from treatment. I have concluded that Theo's progress has plateaued; he has allowed his CFS to define him and limit his potential to find personal fulfillment.

JJ and Deb

When I met JJ, he was ambivalent about the need for treatment. Deb, JJ's wife, insisted that he seek treatment, but when I met the couple, it was clear that JJ was there solely to placate Deb. JJ barely spoke, but I learned he worked at a local hospital. Deb worked at the same hospital in the admissions department. They had no children and had no clear plan to work on her infertility. Both JJ and Deb struggled with obesity.

Prior to his treatment, JJ displayed passive personality traits. He had always struggled in school and had problems with attention and learning. He muddled his way through college but was chronically depressed. His weight gain started in his early 20s, precipitated by one of the medications he was given for depression. By the time I met him, he was well over 300 pounds and gaining more every year. He seemed to be in a serene relationship with Deb; she was doting and attentive, and he was appreciative of her can-do attitude. I pressed him hard to come up with some goals or life objectives. He thought about it for a minute, looked at Deb, and looked back at me. He could not generate an answer.

In addition to obesity, JJ had long-standing fatigue, narcolepsy, and chronic migraines. He had started a medical workup (at Deb's behest) and no clear cause of his fatigue or pain was identified. In the next few weeks, he allowed me to complete the evaluation. I concluded that JJ had CFS. I devised a comprehensive treatment plan involving behavioral therapy and centering on the wakefulness-promoting drug, modafinil.

When I assess the effectiveness of a medication, I use three basic categories to determine its overall effect: mildly effective, moderately effective, or extremely effective. JJ's response to modafinil was in the third category. Within a few weeks of starting medications, JJ hit a stride. His focus and concentration improved. His energy level normalized. The medication decreased JJ's appetite, but more importantly, he adopted disciplined eating habits and daily exercise. His weight dropped precipitously, and within 15 months, his BMI was within the normal range.

Good things started to happen to JJ at work. He was promoted quickly, and within six months, he was in charge of his department. A year later, he enrolled in an MBA program, and before graduation, he was offered a supervisory post in the hospital.

At every turn, JJ found success, and he developed sophisticated ways of defining himself. Soon I realized that his relationship with Deb also changed. He started attending appointments without her and expressed his dissatisfaction with her. For the first time, JJ announced that he resented Deb's infertility and her unwillingness to do anything about it. JJ made some faint effort at marital therapy, but their marriage was broken by conflict, and it ultimately failed. The poignant twist was that although it was Deb's suggestion that her husband enter treatment, once he achieved success, his plans did not include her.

Some Ideas to Consider to Improve Chronic Fatigue

In earlier chapters, I discussed the benefits that may accrue with the use of stimulants to resolve chronic fatigue, and many individuals have found greater energy with the use of central acting medications. Here are a few other ideas to consider:

- Reconsidering what "exercise" is
- Ask yourself if you are tired or sleepy (no, they are not the same)
- Consider warm water hydrotherapy
- Get some exercise if you feel well enough, but stop before you are tired
- On bad days, give yourself a break

Reconsidering "Exercise"

For many people, exercise means a two-mile run and sixty minutes of yoga. To others, exercise happens when you sweat at Pilates, run the treadmill, or work the weight machine. But for a person with chronic fatigue, particularly someone who has been immobile for some time, exercise may need to be redefined. In these situations, start slow and expect to make small, incremental changes over time. When you are trying to regain fitness, exercise could first include walking to the end of the street and, later that month, walking around the block.

Exercising could include dancing at a comfortable pace to your favorite songs, and it might include walking around outside and looking at birds, with or without binoculars. Exercise need not be regimented or executed in perfect time. Start slow, have realistic expectations, and gently increase your capacity. There need not be a race to full fitness. Do not make the mistake of joining an expensive gym before you have a good idea of how you can use the facility. As you reenter the world of fitness, consistency is more important than exertion. Engaging the services of a recreational specialist or a personal trainer, particularly if they understand CFS, can be a helpful guide to restoring your physical well-being.

Drink More Water!

Most people don't drink enough water, and this unduly taxes their renal and GI systems. Some limit their drinking water because they are fearful of bladder control—sometimes their reticence to drink puts them on the verge of dehydration. Avoid this problem! You don't have to drink eight glasses of water, but most people need at least four to six cups of water (or other fluid) per day. Don't achieve your fluid intake solely by consuming caffeinated or sugary beverages. Water may be boring, but it's usually best for the body. Here's why: water helps you avoid constipation, flushes the bacteria from the bladder, improves digestion, and is good for your skin. Even if you are having an inactive day, you still need water. And if you are having an active day, you likely need *more* water, especially when the temperature soars in the summertime.[1]

Note

1. Heidi Godman, "How Much Water Should You Drink?" Harvard Health Publishing, July 18, 2018, https://www.health.harvard.edu/staying-healthy/how-much-water-should-you-drink (accessed July 25, 2019).

Ask Yourself If You're Tired or Sleepy

Many people, including many physicians, believe that if a person is tired, sleep will be the remedy. Sleepiness is a ubiquitous part of the circadian rhythm; almost everyone feels sleepy at some point during the day, and it usually signals us that it is time to take a nap or prepare for a night's sleep. For the average person, a good sleep resolves their sleepiness. In those with CFS, sleep does not restore the individual, and many people with CFS live their lives feeling perpetually sleepy. Cheryl, a dentist newly diagnosed with CFS, told me, "I could sleep fourteen hours and still feel tired. I sleep enough in terms of hours, but my body always feels worn out."

Sleep and CFS have a complicated relationship, and this topic is further explored in Chapter 10. Throughout the book, methods of countering CFS and sleepiness are addressed. Even if these strategies are optimized, people always ask about their continued use of caffeine. It is an important issue that needs to be considered.

Sometimes small amounts of caffeine, delivered courtesy of Starbucks coffee, Lipton Tea, or the Coca-Cola company, give a needed boost. In general, if you are drinking or craving more than two cups per day, you might be self-medicating for an underlying sleep disorder or CFS. If you cannot limit your intake, a referral to a sleep specialist can be helpful in sorting out the potential issues. Countering these medical conditions with appropriate technologies or medications can bring far greater fatigue relief than even high doses of coffee. On the other hand, limited amounts of caffeine may revive your energy levels. People have been consuming caffeinated beverages for hundreds of years, and moderation is generally a good policy.

Postexertional Malaise: What Is It?

Nearly everyone feels tired and fatigued after exercising more than usual. Postexertional malaise refers to the feeling of exhaustion that people with chronic fatigue experience after they move about (not necessarily exercising) more than is typical for them. They may feel well during the activity, whether it's spending an afternoon at the mall or walking the track at the gym. But for the person with CFS experiencing postexertional malaise, the "crash" negates any of the positive momentum realized during the activity.

Consider Warm Water Hydrotherapy

Some researchers have found that even briefly soaking in a hydrotherapy pool improves symptoms of chronic fatigue. Hydrotherapy might even offer a cardiac boost. In a study published in the *South African Journal of Physiotherapy*, researchers noted that warm water immersion had been found to improve heart rate and heart rate variability (HRV) in healthy subjects. The research team set out to evaluate warm water immersion therapy in healthy subjects and to compare the effects to individuals with CFS. All the subjects were evaluated for HRV, meaning the intervals between heartbeats before and after immersion in the warm water.[1]

The researchers did not find a difference in the heart rates of the subjects with CFS compared to the healthy control group subjects; however, they did uncover a lower HRV in the subjects in the CFS group prior to immersion in the warm water. After the immersion, the CFS subjects had the *same* (normal) levels of HRV as the healthy controls. This may mean that warm water immersion could help to stabilize the HRV of people who have CFS.

Suffice it to say that warm water immersion is pleasing to an aching body. This small study suggests that the benefits of this practice include stabilizing HRV in individuals with CFS. The significance of this cardiac effect on long-term outcomes is dubious, but it reinforces the reasons you might want to hop into a Jacuzzi. Before it can be considered a proven practice, further research is needed with a larger number of subjects.

Chronic Fatigue Syndrome + Undiagnosed ADHD Increases Fatigue Intensity

Some researchers have found that the presence of ADHD, along with CFS and depression increases the intensity of fatigue. It also is linked to an earlier age of onset of CFS. In a Spanish study of 158 subjects with CFS, the researchers retrospectively (going back to childhood experiences) diagnosed ADHD in 47 subjects (30%). Of these subjects, 33 still had ADHD (21% of all the subjects). The researchers found that the ADHD subjects had an earlier age of onset of chronic fatigue syndrome (age 30) than the subjects who did not have ADHD (35 years). The ADHD + CFS group also had higher rates of anxiety and depression. The researchers draw the same conclusion that fuels this book; treatment with medications used to treat ADHD might be helpful in the population of ADHD + CFS patients. This group also had a higher risk for suicide.[1]

Note

1. Naia Sáez-Francás, et al., "Attention-Deficit Hyperactivity Disorder in Chronic Fatigue Syndrome Patients," *Psychiatry Research* 200 (2012): 748–753.

Get Some Exercise—But Stop Early before You Tire

CFS fluctuates in intensity; there are good days and days where you think you can't go on. On the better days, it's best not to try to cram every possible activity into this vanishing window. If you push yourself too hard, you may hasten the inevitable crash. Instead, before you try a new challenge or add an extra task, ask yourself the following questions, and then make an informed choice.

1. Is this activity I am considering something I can take slowly, in case I run out of energy? For example, if you're thinking of walking a few blocks to the store, keep in mind that you also must walk those few blocks back home again. Maybe your goal is doable. But if you are thinking you feel so good that you want to walk a mile to prove you can do it, then reconsider. Take this attitude toward whatever

energy-depleting tasks you are considering by breaking the task down into smaller steps.

2. Am I thinking about doing this activity because I really want to do it? Or is my motivation guilt or frustration? ("I never do anything anymore! I'm so awful.") Ask yourself this question and see what pops into your head. If it appears that you would just like to do this activity, such as having lunch with a friend, then seriously consider it.

3. Am I thinking of saying "no" to this activity because the last time I tried this (assuming it's not a very active activity like ice skating or skydiving), I felt bad afterward? Again, could you break the activity down into steps and try the first one or two steps? Then, if you seem okay, perhaps try one further step of this activity.

Advice from People with CFS

People who have been "in the trenches" and are directly suffering from CFS know how difficult this illness can be, and some of them have offered some advice to their fellow sufferers, which is listed below.

- Stop doing anything that isn't absolutely necessary. Just stop!
- Pace yourself! It's important with this illness. It doesn't matter if your friend can run a mile and you can barely run a few steps. This is not a competition. You need to be able to walk safely before you ever consider running. (And running may not be in the cards for you.)
- Stop worrying so much about what other people think of you. No matter what you do, some people are going to criticize you. They just don't get it, and you can't make them know what this illness is like unless they get it themselves. And you really don't want them to get it. Well, maybe for a day or so.
- On the bad days, give yourself a break. On some days when you feel very weak and unable to do much (or anything), don't try to perform activities that you know you cannot do. Give yourself a break. It's not your fault that you have CFS. It's not anyone else's fault, either. It just is the way things are today. Tomorrow will surely be much better.

This chapter covered some basics about how fatigue affects the lives of people with CFS and some nonpharmacological ways to improve your own fatigue levels. The next chapter covers chronic pain, a frequent problem experienced by most people with CFS.

Note

1. Romy Parker, et al., "The Effects of Warm Water Immersion on Blood Pressure, Heart Rate and Heart Rate Variability in People with Chronic Fatigue Syndrome," *South African Journal of Physiotherapy* 74, n. 1 (August 2018), https://www.ncbi.nlm.nih.gov/pmc/articles /PMC6131699/pdf/SAJP-74-442.pdf (accessed July 24, 2019).

CHAPTER 8

Managing Chronic Pain

These frequent headaches and the muscle throbbing that I feel all over my body are really getting to me—it's like it never ends—and sometimes I feel like I've been rubbed raw with pain. I don't want to take opioid drugs like oxycodone; I know they are dangerous—although sometimes I confess that the risk might be worth it just to get some pain relief. My constant fatigue overwhelms me, but the pain bursts make life unbearable. I wish there was something, anything that could make me feel better and give me my life back again! I really need some help!

These were the words used by Jody, a 45-year-old woman who was referred to me five years after she began complaining of chronic fatigue. Along with her severe fatigue, Jody also suffered from frequent episodes of muscle pain that interfered with her life. The pain is not a sharp pain, as is seen with a sudden bone injury, but rather a slow-burning pain characterized by long episodes of throbbing muscle discomfort. For many patients, the pain is interrupted by periods of relative calm, but when the pain reemerges, it feels as if it had never left. Jody came to me in need of a comprehensive plan for pain relief, and my staff and I tried to put together a treatment plan to meet her needs.

A first step is trying to understand whether the fatigue is caused by a medical condition such as OSA or thyroid disease (as discussed in Chapter 3). A clinician must also assess whether an underlying psychiatric condition such as anxiety or depression is contributing to the pain and fatigue. (See Chapter 4 for a full discussion of anxiety and depression.) I recommend that physicians identify and address underlying problems and prescribe appropriate medication for these problems while encouraging positive behaviors, such as effective sleep hygiene, proper diet, and routine exercise.

The Allure of Opioids

In my clinic, we try to steer our patients away from the use of opioids medications for the chronic pain that is associated with CFS. This class of medications is highly seductive for some users. Opioids attach themselves to the mu and delta receptors in the brain, which subsequently leads to increases in the level of the neurochemical dopamine. It is this mechanism that provides a sense of euphoria as well as the analgesic (painkilling) and antianxiety effects. Opioids can be effectively used during brief periods of intense pain or after surgery, and for thousands of years opioids have miraculously reduced human suffering. For example, morphine, the mother agent from which natural opioids are derived (there are also synthetic opioids), has relieved the agony of battlefield wounds and given comforted to countless patients dying from terminal illness.

To the patient with CFS, opioids are a trap. First, opioids never reverse the underlying cause of pain; they only mask the physical discomfort. Second, opioids dull the senses and confuse the body's ability to self-regulate its temperature. Over time, the exposure to the chronic use of opioids impairs a person's memory and judgment. As cognitive impairment is a core characteristic of CFS, opioids make a bad situation even worse. Finally, opioids uniformly worsen the cardinal problem of fatigue. Patients feel drugged, and in subtle ways, their behaviors change in pernicious ways.

As opiates have both analgesic and anxiolytic properties, they are tempting to use in CFS patients. Even in the absence of pain, opiates may seem useful because they decrease anxiety, a symptom overly abundant among patients with CFS. Anxiety is often treated with benzodiazepine medications such as Xanax (alprazolam), and when benzodiazepines and opioids are mixed together, bad things happen. Taken alone, each medication decreases respirations, but when taken together, the effects are additive, and overdose and accidental deaths can easily occur. In the last few years, public health officials have reported an epidemic of opiate abuse and have identified the concurrent use of benzodiazepines as a major risk for premature death. This national tragedy has compelled doctors to limit the use of opiates for chronic pain management.

How Addiction Begins

If opioids are used over a prolonged period, they lose their early analgesic (painkilling) properties. Early on, myalgia pain usually responds to low doses of opiates, but with longer-term exposure, higher doses are needed. Addiction results when the patient develops a physical dependency on the medications. Once the patient becomes tolerant to introductory doses, physical and emotional symptoms surface in the absence of opioids, and this creates an escalating need for ever-higher doses. An agonizing dance begins between the patient, who needs higher doses to maintain her perceived gains, and the doctor, who becomes wary of prescribing a controlled substance. This tension infects the doctor-patient relationship; in the current anti-opioid era in which we live, doctors often feel forced to stop prescribing the medication abruptly. This action may drive the patient to desperation—sometimes even into the streets in search of heroin and other impure opiate derivatives. Opiate addiction wrecks one's judgment and alters the key relationships in a person's life.

Opioid Book That Explains It All

To better understand America's current and ongoing opioid abuse and addiction problem, I recommend the book *The United States of Opioids: A Prescription for Liberating a Nation in Pain* by attorney Harry Nelson (New York: ForbesBooks, 2019). Nelson offers a comprehensive, thoroughly researched, and intriguing view of the use and misuse of opioids from colonial America to the 21st century, providing solid recommendations for resolving this problem. In addition, Nelson has an intuitive grasp of the issues faced by both patients in pain and their physicians.

Describing the Chronic Pain of CFS

At the beginning of the chapter, I described Jody's predicament. Her pain complaints and experiences are typical for individuals with CFS. The pain is achy, not sharp, and it usually migrates throughout her head, back, neck, and arms. Musculoskeletal pain in the trunk and legs is a common problem among people with CFS, as is jaw tightness and pressure in the middle of the chest. CFS pain is unique. Jody's good friend has had diabetes since childhood, and she developed neuropathy, a type of nerve damage that can cause chronic pain. Her friend visited a physical rehabilitation doctor and received relief with nonopiate medications. But Jody's attempt to seek relief was less successful. The same doctor prescribed many of the same pain medications he had given Jody's friend, and Jody started therapy with high hopes. After several months of failed treatment and growing disappointment, Jody inquired why her friend had found relief with the medications and she had not. Her doctor explained that diabetic neuropathy has a well-delineated pain pathway, whereas the physical discomfort associated with CFS is not well understood. Jody appreciated her doctor's honesty, but she still felt angry and frustrated that there was no obvious solution for her pain.

It's important to understand there is *plenty* of hope for chronic pain sufferers in the United States, and this chapter is all about possible solutions, including medications like antidepressants (some of which are specifically approved for pain conditions like fibromyalgia or diabetic nerve pain), antiseizure medications, and, last, "medical marijuana" each with its own set of pros and cons. The chapter also covers CBD oil, a substance that does not include tetrahydrocannabinol (THC), the component of marijuana that induces euphoria and altered states. Many states have passed legislation allowing the use of medical marijuana, and some states now allow the recreational use of marijuana. On the federal level, marijuana is still illegal, and because many banks are regulated by federal law, marijuana transactions largely remain a cash business. Federal law regarding marijuana is largely ignored in states that have affirmed the use of marijuana, but one should be reminded that in states where medical marijuana is still not legal, possessing the substance continues to place the person at risk.

Stimulant medications can combat pain and fatigue in CFS patients. Chapter 6 extensively reviews this concept, but I have included a sidebar on this issue later in this chapter.

Antidepressants Often Help Counter Chronic Pain

Antidepressants are not just for treating depression. In fact, for years, tricyclic antidepressants (amitriptyline or desipramine) have been used to treat chronic pain caused by fibromyalgia, frequent headaches, and other pain conditions.[1] These medications work on neurotransmitters throughout the spinal cord and the brain and have been proven to dampen chronic pain sensation. It is also true that chronic pain and depression often present together, and it can be a dilemma to determine which is the driving force causing the pain sensation—is it an anatomical injury or the result of a biochemically depressed brain? Even the steadiest, most experienced clinician may have a hard time determining the relative contributions of these two factors. It has been suggested that the pain improves because of the antidepressant effect, but some studies have shown that individuals who have no depression at all still realized pain relief from taking an antidepressant.

There are several major types of antidepressants used to treat chronic pain, including tricyclic antidepressants, SSRIs like fluoxetine (Prozac), and serotonin norepinephrine inhibitors (SNRIs) like duloxetine (Cymbalta). The FDA has specifically approved duloxetine for the treatment of fibromyalgia and diabetic neuropathy.[2] Other antidepressants are not specifically approved for the treatment of pain conditions, but physicians regularly prescribe them off-label.

It's Trial and Error with Antidepressants

One factor that frustrates many patients and their doctors is that antidepressants are unpredictable. When working with infectious agents, a clinician can sample urine or blood cultures to determine the proper medications. The same luxury does not apply to antidepressants, which are often a trial-and-error proposition. Patient A with CFS may respond well to amitriptyline (Elavil), but the same medication may be ineffective for the next patient. Doctors know that antidepressant medications dampen pain sensations and improve sleep quality. It's less clear which of many available antidepressants to choose for an individual. Try a medication and see if it helps. If not, move on to another antidepressant class.

Unlike long-acting stimulants, antidepressants do not significantly enhance energy or concentration, and for this reason, they are less effective overall for CFS pain. Bear in mind that all medications, including antidepressants, carry side effects, and sometimes the "cure" is worse than the underlying problem. At times, the adverse effects of the antidepressant—weight gain, constipation, sedation, and sexual dysfunction—are not worth the potential benefit to the patient. In overdose, tricyclic antidepressants can cause heart rhythm disturbances and even death. Still, antidepressants have been around for decades, and millions of chronic pain patients have gained great relief from these medications. Paul, a 61-year-old teacher with fibromyalgia and chronic fatigue, came to my clinic after having been on a nortriptyline dosage of 25 mg at night. His comments reflect the typical way patients with chronic pain view their antidepressant. "I think it helps me. My nerve pain feels more muted when I take it. I have tried to stop nortriptyline because of constipation, but I return to it because it makes me feel less anxious and I can more easily fall asleep."

Table 8.1 provides a list of the key antidepressants and their possible side effects.

Table 8.1 Antidepressants Used On or Off-Label to Treat Chronic Pain Conditions

Generic (Brand Name)	Types of Chronic Pain Conditions Used For	Possible Side Effects
Tricyclic Antidepressants		
Amitriptyline (Elavil)	Used off-label for chronic headaches	Dry mouth, constipation, weight gain, drowsiness, unsafe in overdose
Desipramine (Norpramin)	Used off-label for neuropathic pain	Dry mouth, constipation, unsafe in overdose
Imipramine (Tofranil)	Used off-label for neuropathic pain	Dry mouth, weakness, diarrhea or constipation, decreased sexual drive, unsafe in overdose
Serotonin Reuptake Inhibitors (SRIs)		
Fluoxetine (Prozac)	May improve irritable bowel syndrome, or chronic low back pain; off-label	Sexual dysfunction, weight gain
Serotonin Norepinephrine Reuptake Inhibitors (SNRIs)		
Duloxetine (Cymbalta)	Approved by FDA for pain of diabetic neuropathy and fibromyalgia; off-label for other forms of chronic pain	Dry mouth, nausea, dizziness, sexual dysfunction, constipation, weight gain
Milnacipran (Savella)	Approved by the FDA for fibromyalgia pain	Dry mouth, nausea, dizziness, sexual dysfunction, constipation, weight gain
Venlafaxine (Effexor)	Off-label for migraine headaches	Sexual dysfunction and withdrawal effects if medication is stopped abruptly

(continued)

Table 8.1 (*continued*)

Generic (Brand Name)	Types of Chronic Pain Conditions Used For	Possible Side Effects
Other Antidepressants		
Bupropion (Wellbutrin, Wellbutrin XL)	Off-label for neuropathic pain	Agitation, dry mouth, headache, insomnia, nausea and vomiting

Sources: Raphael J. Leo and Khalid, Kiran, "Antidepressants for Chronic Pain," *Current Psychiatry* 18, n. 2 (February 2019): 9–22; Carina Riediger, et al. "Adverse Effects of Antidepressants for Chronic Pain: A Systematic Review and Meta-Analysis," *Frontiers in Neurology* 8, n. 307 (July 2017): 1–23, https://www.ncbi.nlm.nih.gov/pmc/articles/PMC5510574/pdf/fneur-08-00307.pdf; American Academy of Neurology, "Study Finds Bupropion SR Effective in Treating Neuropathic Pain," November 12, 2001, https://www.aan.com/PressRoom/Home/PressRelease/105 (accessed March 22, 2019); Aisha Morris Moultry and Poon, Ivy O., "The Use of Antidepressants for Chronic Pain," May 9, 2009, https://www.uspharmacist.com/article/the-use-of-antidepressants-for-chronic-pain (accessed March 22, 2019).

General Advice for Consumers on Antidepressants

Several considerations dictate the use of antidepressant medications for chronic pain:

1. Start low and go slow. Because the antidepressant is being used for pain control rather than depression, one can start with a lower dosage. If sufficient relief is not gained at a low dosage, a higher dosage may be needed to determine if the medication is helpful.
2. Keep in mind that some drugs take a while to gain full strength. Antidepressants are not narcotics, and they will not provide precipitous pain relief. Some antidepressants may take weeks to reach a full effect.
3. Do not assume that if one antidepressant offers no pain relief, all antidepressants are worthless for pain control. In these situations, a trial with another antidepressant from another class is in order.
4. Do not expect complete resolution of all pain sensations. Look for trends in improvements; early pain relief generally heralds longer-term success.

Antiseizure Medications

Another category of medication commonly used to treat chronic pain is the anticonvulsants, a class of medication originally designed to treat epilepsy. These medications are often used off-label to treat chronic pain, especially neuropathic (nerve) pain. Gabapentin (Neurontin) is used for neuropathic pain, as is lamotrigine (Lamictal). Pregabalin (Lyrica), the newest drug in this class, is widely researched in pain conditions. All these medications may be sedating and should be used carefully.

In a meta-analysis published in 2011, researchers reviewed 12 studies of lamotrigine for both acute and chronic pain. The pain conditions included in the study were diabetic neuropathy, neuropathic pain, spinal cord injury-related pain, and other types of sharp pain experienced by adults. In diabetic neuropathy, some studies with lamotrigine showed a 20–50 percent reduction in pain intensity. The main adverse event was a problem with skin rash, experienced by 10 percent of the lamotrigine group compared to 6 percent of the placebo group.[3]

Anticonvulsants hold appeal because they are proven to work in diabetic neuropathy, and in contrast to opioids, they have little addictive potential. These medications work less well for chronic generalized pain, and overall, anticonvulsants play a limited role for the CFS/ME patient.

Stimulants for CFS Pain

Stimulants can play a role in treating chronic pain. The process is complicated, but basically, chronic pain may be associated with a burnout of various neurochemicals throughout the brain. People with chronic pain often have low levels of natural chemicals called catecholamines, such as epinephrine, norepinephrine, and dopamine. This relative deficit leads to a dulled nervous system and accentuated pain levels. Prescribed stimulant medications act as catecholamines, effectively reversing this deficit and decreasing pain.[1] Some patients relate that stimulants provide pain relief that is equivalent to that of opioids.[2] The use of a stimulant in a person with chronic pain may have an effect similar to a car with a stalled battery: it recharges the battery, and the car (or person) is ready to function normally (or better) again.

Notes

1. Forest Tennant, "Status Report on Role of Stimulants in Chronic Pain Management," *Practical Pain Management* n. 6 (2015), https://www.practicalpain management.com/treatments/pharmacological/non-opioids/status-report -role-stimulants-chronic-pain-management (accessed May 1, 2019).

2. Ibid.

Medical Marijuana or CBD OIL: Pros and Cons

Medical marijuana is prescribed to individuals with severe and chronic pain. Prescriptions are often granted to cancer patients as well as those who suffer from glaucoma, fibromyalgia, and other pain syndromes. The legality of medical marijuana differs widely; some states strictly regulate it while others exert little control. Neighboring states may have completely different laws; recreational marijuana is legal in Colorado but is not lawful in the bordering state of Wyoming.

As of this writing, 10 states have legalized the recreational use of marijuana among adults, including Alaska, California, Colorado, Maine, Massachusetts, Michigan, Nevada, Oregon, Vermont, and Washington (as well as Washington, D.C.). In addition, 34 states, plus the District of Columbia, Guam, and Puerto Rico, have laws regarding the use of medical marijuana (cannabis).[4] The number of states liberalizing marijuana laws will continue to grow, and there does not seem to be significant effort from the medical community opposing this social policy change. As the practice is so widespread, it is appropriate to offer an overview about the current understanding of marijuana and cannabidiol (CBD) as they relate to chronic pain conditions.

Medical Marijuana: Does It Play a Role?

Even medical experts who prescribe medical marijuana disagree on the wisdom of widespread adoption of marijuana as a treatment for pain. Some physicians argue that marijuana should be legalized nationwide, whereas other doctors, sometimes within the same practice or university, believe that marijuana use poses a serious problem. I am a skeptic regarding the role of marijuana in chronic pain management.

Some Young Adults Use Marijuana to Treat Chronic Pain

Although many people perceive medical marijuana as a drug that may ease the pain of terminal disease, a study of 143 young adults who regularly used marijuana revealed that 40 percent used the drug for chronic pain. The pain was primarily musculoskeletal, abdominal, and migraine/headache pain. This rate is surprising because it is double the previous estimates of chronic pain in young adults.[1]

A deeper dive reveals interesting ways young people use marijuana. The subjects with chronic pain had a higher percentage of heavy marijuana users compared to those who did not report pain. For example,

5 percent of the people in the chronic pain group used marijuana daily, which is five times the rate of the subjects without chronic pain. Chronic pain users were also more likely to use the drug while alone (51%) compared to the subjects without pain (21%).[2] It appears that the subjects who were not in pain were interested in using marijuana to promote sociability rather than for its analgesic properties. Finally, the researchers found that those who used marijuana for pain used a greater quantity of the drug at each use.

We typically think of young adults as vibrant and healthy beings, yet the study reveals that some in this group suffers from chronic pain at alarmingly high rates. Although the study did not delineate whether any of these young adults had CFS, it seems likely that CFS was represented in the study; still, further exploration is warranted. Clinicians must balance marijuana research findings that show positive effects with the knowledge that marijuana clouds the senses and impairs cognitive clearness. The payoff may be too high a price to pay for young people in the most dynamic phase of their scholastic life.

Notes

1. Jessica L. Fales, Ladd, Benjamin O., and Magnan, Renee E., "Pain Relief as a Motivation for Cannabis Use among Young Adult Users with and without Chronic Pain," *Journal of Pain* (2019), https://doi.org/1016/j.pain.2019.02.001 (accessed April 30, 2019).

2. Ibid.

Insufficient Evidence for the Types of Marijuana That People Actually Use

Many anecdotal claims are made regarding marijuana's impact on pain. Marijuana has been promoted as a drug that improves both acute cancer pain and chronic intermittent conditions, such as low back pain, neuropathic (nerve) pain, inflammatory pain, and the pain associated with migraine headaches. Despite the hype, there is a surprising lack of scientific evidence to fortify these claims, largely because until recently, investigators had trouble accessing regulated marijuana for controlled research. There are exceptions; a few prescribed forms of marijuana are approved by the FDA for research treating cancer pain, epilepsy, and other specific pain syndromes. In the next few years, more research will emerge from public and private sectors, trying to clarify the role of marijuana in treating pain.

Although the FDA is expressing openness to proper marijuana research, another part of the federal government, the DEA, emits different signals. To the DEA, marijuana has always been considered an illegal substance, but in 2013, the agency announced that it would defer the right to challenge marijuana legalization laws in the states that have approved medical marijuana.[5]

So does marijuana improve chronic pain? Penny Whiting and colleagues have concluded that marijuana does improve some pain conditions. Her team analyzed 28 studies of medical marijuana, of which 13 studies were for chronic pain. Smoked or vaporized THC was used in five of the 13 cases. The subjects had widely varying types of chronic pain, including cancer pain, diabetic neuropathy, fibromyalgia, rheumatoid arthritis, and other forms of pain. The researchers found that pain reduction was significantly higher in the cannabinoid group compared to the placebo group.[6] Whiting concluded, "There was moderate-quality evidence to support the use of cannabinoids for the treatment of chronic pain and spasticity."[7]

Another analysis of 24 clinical trials examined cannabis-based medicines for managing pain, particularly neuropathic pain. The researchers determined there was "limited evidence" of efficaciousness. The studies were imperfectly executed, as nearly all the studies were limited to one dosage of the drug, and only a few studies examined inhalation, the means by which most people use the marijuana.[8]

Significant side effects were evident from marijuana use, such as diarrhea, dry mouth, heartburn, mouth ulceration, and vomiting. In addition, psychological adverse events were reported, including confusion, anxiety, hallucinations, paranoia, racing thoughts, unpleasant dreams, and increased appetite. Some studies reported visual adverse effects such as blurred vision or a change in vision, while a few noted the development of tinnitus or vertigo.[9] It should also be noted that marijuana can trigger psychotic reactions, and it is impossible to assess in advance which people are vulnerable to this catastrophic side effect.[10]

The National Academy of Sciences has reported on clinical studies using FDA-approved forms of marijuana for patients with cancer or other extremely severe illnesses and found that patients did gain some pain relief. The report that relied largely on Whiting's research concluded, "There is substantial evidence that cannabis is an effective treatment for chronic pain in adults."[11] This letter of encouragement from such a prestigious organization has intensified commercial and research interest in marijuana.

Some States Approve Marijuana as Treatment for Opioid Addiction

The mind-set about marijuana in many states in the United States has changed dramatically and quickly, based on changes in state laws. Whereas the safety concerns about of marijuana for recreational use are unresolved, and experts are still trying to capture its proper use as a medical therapeutic, some advocate that marijuana is an unequivocal positive force. The states of Illinois, New Jersey, New York, and Pennsylvania have approved the use of marijuana as a treatment option for those using or abusing opioids. For example, in New Jersey, "opioid use disorder" was added to other conditions for which marijuana use became lawful. Among the most notable skeptics of this practice is Nora Volkow, MD, director of the National Institute of Drug Abuse. In 2019, Volkow expressed concern that people addicted to heroin, OxyContin, and other opioids will self-administer marijuana instead of pursuing FDA-approved treatment drugs such as buprenorphine, methadone, and naltrexone. Volkow asserts that there is no scientific evidence to support marijuana as a treatment for opioid addiction in 2019.[1]

This concern is justified; the use of marijuana to overcome an opioid addiction is a dangerous and potentially life-threatening path. Instead, individuals addicted to opioids should seek medical attention from experienced physicians who can offer psychological and, if needed, pharmacological support to help curb addiction. Withdrawal from opioids often requires medical supervision, and once this detoxification is in process, addiction risk factors such as anxiety, depression, ADHD, and chronic pain and fatigue need to be addressed in a biopsychosocial model that considers all these aspects to minimize the risk of substance use relapse.

Note

1. Ken Alltucker, "Marijuana as a Cure for Opioid Use? Nation's Top Drug Scientists Says She's Skeptical," *USA Today*, March 20, 2019, https://www.usatoday.com /story/news/health/2019/03/20/weed-marijuana-cannabis-opioid-addiction -withdrawal-nida-nora-volkow/3221792002/ (accessed May 1, 2019).

I worry that medical marijuana has been adopted before there has been enough study to justify its casual use. Over the years, the FDA has developed elaborate methods to test the safety and efficacy of prescribed over-the-counter medications. This agency maintains high standards, and all Americans rely on their approval process to ensure our families have safe foods and drugs. It is strange indeed that the FDA has not been given jurisdiction over medical marijuana. No other comprehensive safety oversight has been put in its place, and I am concerned that the lack of good regulation puts citizens at risk. In the marijuana industry's haste to legitimize their products, I fear that we have subverted our well-developed public health protections.

As a result of not having appropriate oversight, consumers may not know the amount of the marijuana they ingest (although some states provide labeling of dosages of THC). In addition, the potency of marijuana today is far greater than it was in past decades. We are not yet certain how marijuana interacts with other medications or how it affects health conditions such as heart disease or diabetes. There is not enough data to determine whether marijuana is safe in pregnancy or nursing. There is peril with adopting treatments too quickly. In the 1960s, the drug thalidomide was given to pregnant women with morning sickness, and this drug resulted in devastating birth defects in their female children. (A forward-thinking American doctor at the FDA banned the use of thalidomide in the United States, preventing many tragedies.[12]) Without extensive FDA involvement and oversight, this type of tragedy could strike again.

Marijuana That Is Approved by the Feds

The FDA has approved several drugs that contain either marijuana or cannabidiol (CBD) to treat some specific medical problems. For example, in 2018, the medication Epidolex, which includes CBD as its active ingredient, was approved to treat some patients with severe seizures caused by epilepsy. The medication dronabinol (Syndros) was approved by the FDA in 2016 to treat two conditions: severe weight loss caused by acquired immune deficiency syndrome (AIDS) and nausea and vomiting resulting from cancer chemotherapy regimens. Nabilone (Cesamet) and dronabinol (Marinol), two synthetic THC drugs, were approved in 1985 to treat nausea and vomiting that was induced by cancer chemotherapy.[1] It is also important to note that these drugs are in pill form because researchers were not able to allow smoked, vaped, or edible marijuana in their studies.

Note

1. Karen Hande, "Cannabidiol," *Supportive Care* 23, n. 2 (April 2019): 131–134.

Cannabidiol (CBD)

The key difference between marijuana and CBD is that CBD does not contain THC, the ingredient in marijuana that leads to the sensation of being high. CBD comes from the hemp plant, which is related to the marijuana plant, or *cannabis sativa*. Marijuana also contains CBD, as well as many other chemical components.

Cannabidiol generally refers to cannabis oil. It is an item that is available in most states and online, and the claims for its efficacy in pain management range from mild support to wild enthusiasm. It has been suggested for countless conditions; one can find a web page claiming that CBD is effective in psoriasis, male-pattern baldness, and acne. Peter Grinspoon, MD, cited studies indicating that CBD may improve neuropathic (nerve) pain and inflammatory pain. CBD may also play a role in the management of insomnia and anxiety. Grinspoon cautions that CBD should not be taken concurrently with warfarin (Coumadin) because it could cause an increase in the warfarin blood levels.[13] (Warfarin is a blood thinner, and it would be dangerous for the blood to become too thin.)

Dr. Grinspoon also voices concern about CBD product labeling. CBD is sold under the lax federal supplement laws governing drugs like melatonin and chamomile. For that reason, the appropriate dosages for CBD have not yet been delineated. Still, hype should never surpass skepticism, and it would be preferable for CBD to be subjected to the higher FDA standard that oversee over-the-counter painkilling drugs like acetaminophen (Tylenol) or ibuprofen and, of course, prescribed medications.

As CBD does not cross the barrier into the brain, it does not generate euphoria or any sort of high in the user. (If it does, then the drug probably contains THC.) As true CBD never enters the brain, many doctors are skeptical that it offers any true or lasting benefit. It is suspected that many individuals who take CBD benefit from the "placebo effect," which occurs when subjects are given a sugar pill rather than a treatment drug. Because people believe that they are taking a "real" drug, it is this belief not the properties of an active drug that offers them relief. The placebo effect isn't necessarily a bad thing, but it eventually wears off when real pain asserts itself. A true test of a treatment is whether patients refill the medication. With CBD, they usually do not (see Tables 8.2 and 8.3 for a discussion of the pros and cons of using marijuana and CBD oil for chronic pain).

Table 8.2 The Pros and Cons of Using Marijuana for Chronic Pain

Pros	Cons
• Marijuana may provide pain relief.	• Marijuana may cause mental slowness and memory impairment. Frequent and regular use has a negative impact on motivation.
• Marijuana may be easy to obtain.	• A state may have many restrictive rules and regulations about the use of marijuana.
• Marijuana use may give a person a chance to reclaim her life from pain.	• Smoking marijuana can cause damage to the lungs and throat, and other forms of the drug may be unavailable. Also, smoked marijuana may include harmful substances, as does tobacco. Sometimes marijuana is adulterated with dangerous fillers.
• Other medications may have failed to provide pain relief, but marijuana may provide such relief.	• The quality and purity of marijuana can vary, especially when a person is obtaining the substance from unreliable sources.
• Increasing numbers of people/states have begun to be much more favorable toward marijuana use for pain control.	• Person will test positive for marijuana on a drug screen for employment or other purposes. Even though government is moving toward legalization, many private employers maintain polices forbidding marijuana.
• Marijuana offers a sense of well-being to individuals suffering from anxiety and depression.	• Some researchers have found that regular marijuana use may induce psychotic features in select individuals.
• Marijuana use has become destigmatized, even encouraged, in adolescents.	• The drug is dangerous for adolescents with chronic pain because it negatively impacts cognitive function and motivation.

A Concern with CBD Oil: Product Labeling and Safety

Some organizations have tested random samples of CBD products and found that in many cases, the contents of the drug were very different from what was promised on the label. For example, in a detailed letter to the *Journal of the American Medical Association*, researchers reported purchasing and testing 84 items that purportedly contained CBD. They subsequently tested these items and found that less than half (45%) of the items were accurately labeled. In addition, they also found the presence of unreported THC in 21 percent of the samples; THC is an illegal substance in such products, and the levels of THC that they identified may have been enough to induce impairment, particularly if a child took the drug accidentally (or purposely). They concluded that additional monitoring was needed for these products.[1]

Note

1. Marcel O. Bonn-Miller, et al., "Research Letter: Labeling Accuracy of Cannabidiol Extracts Sold Online," *Journal of the American Medical Association* 318, n. 2 (November 7, 2017): 1708–1709.

Table 8.3 Pros and Cons of Using CBD Oil for Chronic Pain

Pros	Cons
• CBD does not contain THC, the euphoric ingredient in marijuana, which causes sedation, euphoria, and lack of concentration.	• CBD does not have THC, the euphoric/sedating ingredient in marijuana (THC may be needed to combat pain).
• CBD oils are rubbed into the skin and specifically not inhaled.	• It can be difficult to know what the correct dosage is, and the manufacturer is not always a reliable source because of less strict federal rules governing supplements.
• CBD may give some pain relief.	• CBD may be ineffective. Pain relief may be a placebo effect. • Interactions with other medications a possibility.
• Person may believe the CBD works, so it does work—for a while.	• Person may test positive for marijuana in a drug screen for employment or other purposes.

A Psychiatrist's General Advice for Consumers Considering Medical Marijuana or CBD

This chapter sets forth the arguments for and against using medical marijuana and CBD for chronic pain associated with CFS. Although I am not hiding my skepticism, I am stopping short of taking an entrenched position. I do realize that many experts take a different view, and I respect all good arguments. On this position, everyone needs to make informed decisions for themselves and for their families. A few summary points:

1. Make sure you understand the laws in your state about medical marijuana and/or CBD. State laws vary drastically, and although in some states, you may be able to grow a small number of marijuana plants, that possession could get you a jail sentence in other states. You may be required to buy the marijuana or CBD from a state-regulated licensed facility.
2. Do not assume that laws in a neighboring state will be like the ones in your home state. Always check first. Also, if you legally buy marijuana in one state, do not assume you can transport it home to your own state.
3. If you obtain marijuana or CBD, use only a small quantity the first time so that you can see how the drug affects you. Start low and go slow.
4. Don't plan on driving after you use the marijuana or CBD. The drug may impede or impair your driving ability. Some states have "driving while drugged" laws, which are like driving while intoxicated (DWI) with alcohol. Marijuana can't be breath-tested, but it can be tested for in the blood or urine. For example, in Colorado, if a driver's blood tests positive for THC in quantities of 5 mg/ml or greater, then it may be assumed that the driver was under the influence of marijuana.[14]
5. Never assume that the pain reduction a friend has with marijuana or CBD will be similar to yours. Drugs and medications affect different people differently.
6. In these uncharted waters, one thing is clear: marijuana negatively affects mental clarity and can alter perception, judgment, memory, and physical coordination.[15] Marijuana also has an abuse and addiction potential, and about 9 percent of adult users develop an addiction. If the drug is initially used in adolescence, the addiction risk nearly doubles to 17 percent.[16] This is a steep price to pay—even for relief from CFS-associated chronic pain.

Notes

1. Raphael J. Leo and Kirens Khalid, "Antidepressants for Chronic Pain," *Current Psychiatry* 18, n. 2 (February 2019): 9–22.

2. Ibid.

3. Philip J. Wiffen, Derry, Sheena, and Moore, R. Andrew, "Lamotrigine for Acute and Chronic Pain," *Cochrane Database Systems Review*, 2011, https://www.cochranelibrary.com/cdsr/doi/10.1002/14651858.CD0 06044.pub3/epdf/full (accessed May 1, 2019).

4. National Conference of State Legislatures, "Drugged Driving/Marijuana-Impaired Driving," March 8, 2019, http://www.ncsl .org/research/transportation/drugged-driving-overview.aspx (accessed March 22, 2019).

5. National Conference of State Legislatures, "State Medical Marijuana Laws," March 5, 2019, http://www.ncsl.org/research/health/state -medical-marijuana-laws.aspx (accessed March 22, 2019).

6. Penny F. Whiting, et al., "Cannabinoids for Medical Use: A Systematic Review and Meta-Analysis," *Journal of the American Medical Association* 313, n. 24 (2015): 2456–2473.

7. Ibid., page 2456.

8. J. Aviram and Samuelly-Leichtag, G., "Efficacy of Cannabis-Based Medicines for Pain Management: A Systematic Review and Meta-Analysis of Randomized Controlled Trials," *Pain Physician* 20 (2017), https://www.painphysicianjournal.com/current/pdf?article=NDYwNA %3D%3D&journal=107 (accessed March 22, 2019).

9. Ibid.

10. Deepak Cyril O'Souza and Ranganathan, Mohini, "Medical Marijuana: Is the Cart before the Horse?" *Journal of the American Medical Association* 313, n. 24 (June 23–30, 2015): 2431–2432.

11. National Academies of Sciences, Engineering, and Medicine. *The Health Effects of Cannabis and Cannabinoids: The Current States of Evidence and Recommendations for Research*. Washington, DC: The National Academies Press, 2017, page 90.

12. Robert D. McFadden, "Frances Oldham Kelsey, Who Saved U.S. Babies from Thalidomide, Dies at 101," *New York Times,* August 7, 2015, https://www.nytimes.com/2015/08/08/science/frances-oldham-kelsey -fda-doctor-who-exposed-danger-of-thalidomide-dies-at-101.html (accessed May 2, 2019).

13. Peter Grinspoon, "Cannabidiol (CBD)—What We Know and What We Don't," *Harvard Health blog, Harvard Medical School,* August 24, 2018, https://www.health.harvard.edu/blog/cannabidiol-cbd

-what-we-know-and-what-we-dont-2018082414476 (accessed May 2, 2019).

14. National Conference of State Legislatures, "Drugged Driving /Marijuana-Impaired Driving," March 8, 2019, http://www.ncsl.org /research/transportation/drugged-driving-overview.aspx (accessed March 22, 2019).

15. Richard J. Schrot and Hubbard, John R., "Cannabinoids: Medical Implications," *Annals of Medicine* 48, n. 3 (2016): 128–141.

16. Ibid.

CHAPTER 9

Brain Fog: What It Is and How You Can Gain Relief

Nora used to figure out restaurant charges with ease, and she was the person who could factor in the tip and split the charges. Her friends knew her as someone who could engage in witty conversation, and her direct comebacks always made people laugh. Over the last few years, Nora felt none of her previous sharpness. Words did not flow as easily, and she had trouble recalling the names of people she had recently met. Most of the time she felt fatigued and dull. "It's like living through a giant cotton ball that wads up my thoughts. I feel like a major dummy, so different than the way I used to feel about myself." Nora is 35, much too young for Alzheimer's disease, and her doctors have assured her that she does not have an infection, a brain tumor, or an autoimmune process. After five years of suffering with the draining symptoms, Nora has learned that she has CFS. She wonders what causes her symptoms. "If it took me so long to get a diagnosis, what are other patients like me being told?" Finally, Nora asks what she can do to improve her thinking.

Nora's experience reflects the brain fog of CFS. This is the descriptive phrase used throughout the book, and it should be defined. Brain fog connotes difficulty in thinking, reacting, planning, organizing, remembering, concentrating, and performing. Psychologists refer to these properties as "executive" abilities. Every healthy adult has some level of executive functioning; however, people who have CFS, and specifically the subgroup of CFS patients who have brain fog, notice a decline of their executive abilities. Understanding and dealing with executive dysfunction is a great mystery of the CFS story.

Think of the healthiest and brightest person you know. Let's call her Alice Amazing, and imagine that as Alice enters her mid-30s, she develops severe exhaustion and persistent body pain. No matter how many hours she sleeps, she still feels tired and dull. There is no chance that she will be able to sustain her high level of functioning. Alice Amazing has become, at least for now, Alice Below-Average. Previous chapters cover other aspects of CFS, medication approaches (Chapter 6), resolving severe fatigue (Chapter 7), and chronic pain (Chapter 8). Chapter 10 concerns problems with sleep in CFS. I contend that once these other symptoms are addressed, brain fog will improve considerably. This chapter explains the brain effects of CFS and focuses on methods to reverse brain fog.

People with CFS frequently have impaired working memory and concentration. In a study that compared patients with combined CFS and fibromyalgia (43 subjects) to patients with CFS alone (50 subjects), researchers found that the combined group had more cognitive complaints and were slower to complete tasks than the patients with CFS alone. Furthermore, the combined group had a poorer performance than the CFS-alone group on norms for tasks of verbal memory and visual-perceptual ability. Finally, the combined group realized clinical improvement at a slower rate than did the patients with only CFS.[1]

Unfortunately, this study did not contain a control group, but the most compelling finding is that both groups performed below the expected norm for healthy individuals who had neither condition.[2] These cognitive functions constitute brain fog and are controlled by the cerebral cortex and associated brain structures. It is safe to say that brain fog is indeed "in your head"; all these brain-based activities constitute real functional impairment that interferes with personal contentment.

The medical community has tried to understand brain fog associated with CFS. In his detailed report in *Frontiers in Physiology*, physiologist Anthony J. Ocon defines brain fog as confusion, slowed thinking, hazy thought processes, forgetfulness, and a lack of concentration. Ocon also notes that children with CFS have been found to have impaired working memory and auditory learning as well as a limited ability to switch their attention from one task to another. Ocon asserts that these symptoms result from decreased cerebral blood flow throughout the brain, a condition referred to as postural tachycardia syndrome (POTS).[3] In the POTS model, the weak and fluctuating blood perfusion underpowers the brain, which results in the clinical manifestation of brain fog.[4]

As I have relayed in earlier chapters, I suspect that many cases of CFS are the result of childhood ADHD. Ocon's description of brain fog uses many of the same words other experts use to describe features of ADHD. Ocon suggests that inadequate blood perfusion into the brain causes brain fog. In contrast, I believe that brain fog results from the same biological process that causes ADHD, namely a complex dysregulation of the brain's dopamine and norepinephrine modulation. Chapter 5 offers evidence that treating CFS/brain fog with long-acting stimulant medications, the mainstay of ADHD treatment, ameliorates cognitive symptoms. Explaining brain fog as a result of hypoperfusion or as a function of the natural history of ADHD is a prime example of two observers describing the same clinical problem but deriving vastly different conceptualizations about cause and then treatment.

Through this chapter, I have cited many studies to demonstrate the varied thinking about brain fog and to emphasize that there is no consensus about its causes. All experts do agree that brain fog is a core part of the spectrum of symptoms that make up CFS. This chapter is about working with this problem and, whenever possible, making it better.

Brain Fog Is Powerful

"Brain fog completely affects me and controls my life because I cannot think clearly at all. Most of the time I feel like I am in a dream, even though I know this is my true life. It just feels so foggy. Some times are worse than others, but it never fully goes away. I'm angry that I can't remember anyone's name."

The Elements of Brain Fog

It's important to break down the key elements of brain fog and to realize that patients experience these symptoms with varying intensity and proportion, no two the same. Here's a list of the most common symptoms:

• Difficulty with concentration
• Difficulty making plans
• Problems with recall

- Inability to follow through on plans
- Lack of motivation to do "all of the above"

Difficulty with Concentration

It can be extremely frustrating for a person with brain fog to concentrate on listening to another person or performing a task that requires concentration. Yet there are a myriad of tasks that present every day, from preparing a meal to learning new business software, to reviewing a child's homework, to planning a family vacation. The person with CFS may have trouble concentrating because she is poorly organized or preoccupied with feelings of distress.

Difficulty Making Plans

Even something as routine as going to a grocery store requires a plan. For most people this mundane task is an intuitive reflex—not so for individuals with executive dysfunction. Consider the planning and organization that goes into a shopping trip. To begin, a list needs to be generated (after an inventory of the pantry is taken). The list must be placed in one's wallet, and there must be gas in the car for the drive to the supermarket. Once at the store, the shopper needs to locate the items, wait for the cashier, bag the merchandise, put the bags in a cart, leave the store, put the bags in the car, and drive home. Once home, the bags need to be unloaded and placed in the appropriate place. Sounds simple, right?

Yet for a person who has trouble making or executing a plan, there are so many ways for this exercise to go wrong. You might forget to make a list. You must search for your car keys (I wish I always put the keys in the same place when I'm done using them). At the store, you cannot recall what tonight's recipe calls for. You walk out of the store, leaving one of the bags on the counter. This time someone who works at the market notices your forgotten bag and runs after you with the package that you place behind the driver's seat. Back at home, you remember to carry the bags from the garage into the kitchen but then notice that the cupboards are a mess (you forgot to organize them last weekend), and there is no place to store the new groceries. You realize, "Damn I bought another bottle of maple syrup. I didn't know that I had two unopened bottles." Or, you could jump through all these hoops until the next morning when you notice the butter pecan ice cream you forgot to unload is a melted puddle in the backseat of your new car.

Problems with Recall

People with brain fog complain that their recall fails them at inopportune moments. You forget the name of your colleague's children or the name of the person you met 30 seconds ago at a party. Your spouse asks you to retrieve something from the basement, but when you get there, you can't remember what was requested. It's that hazy feeling in your brain again, and it's blurring away the sharp edges of a clear mind, dulling it and dumbing it down. This frustrating feeling is a common characteristic of brain fog among people with CFS.

Inability to Follow Through

Another part of brain fog is the difficulty a person has with following through on a plan. You wanted to file your expense report, but somehow you got sidetracked by another office project. You fully intended to pay your son's college tuition so that he did not have trouble registering for the new semester, but you never got around to it. Sometimes you can recover in time and correct yourself; other times, the inability to follow through means that you missed a hard deadline, and now the Delta flight to Orlando has tripled in price.

Lack of Motivation

The brain fog of CFS may also infect a person with a chronic lack of motivation. What does it all matter anyway? Who cares if your report is late—what's the big deal? But it is a big deal. When a person is not motivated enough to perform important tasks, then others will stop relying on him. He will be seen as undependable and someone who cannot be counted on to do anything right. Once this reputation is solidified, future opportunities dry up.

Motivated people do their homework on time and study for tests in advance. They turn in their college applications before the deadline and go the extra yard to impress their employer. Without motivation, it is hard to save for the future, exercise preventative health behaviors, and even make sure your hair is combed and there is no kale in your teeth. Impaired motivation is one of the core features of brain fog and may be the symptom that is most impairing.

It is important to keep in mind that, sadly, CFS is often stigmatized by others. Sometimes even doctors perceive people with CFS as lazy individuals who don't want to work and who would prefer to be cared for by other people. This stigma can be prominent, and it is very painful for people with CFS.

When Brain Fog Is a Key Symptom: Other Brain Diseases to Consider

CFS is not the only disorder in which cognitive impairment is a dominant symptom, and because of this, people who present to physicians with concerns of poor memory, lack of concentration, and impaired motivation may be evaluated for other brain diseases. Do not be surprised if your doctor attempts to rule out these major diagnoses, which may include early-onset Alzheimer's disease (for people younger than age 65), vascular dementia, mild cognitive impairment (MCI), and chronic traumatic encephalopathy (CTE).

The symptoms of brain fog within the context of CFS look alarmingly like early dementia or brain injury. Doctors need to integrate this understanding into their practice because CFS and related conditions, in distinction to the dementias, are readily treatable conditions. If the CFS diagnosis is overlooked, the patient is deprived of a meaningful treatment option. The next section offers a brief discussion of neurological conditions that are frequently confused with CFS conditions and provides a table comparing these diagnoses.

Brain Fog versus Dementia

Amelia came to our clinic because she was distressed over her memory loss and profound fatigue. Her sadness took root after she was diagnosed with "early Alzheimer's" by a neurologist who met with her twice. "I can't bear the thought of losing my mind," she told me. "My mother-in-law died from Alzheimer's, and at the end, she could not feed herself or do anything for herself."

I suspected that the diagnosis of dementia was not accurate for a number or reasons. Amelia was 65 years old, a young, but not unheard-of age for someone to develop dementia. She also had a good sense of humor and related well to me and my staff. She spoke well and was wearing fashionable clothes. I interviewed her carefully and spoke with her family to get a full background of Amelia's recent functioning.

Amelia was concerned that it took her a while to remember certain information. I asked her to clarify this complaint, and she demonstrated to me that she knew the names of her grandchildren and where they were going to college. She was distressed that she often forgot the time she promised to meet her husband for dinner. When pressed, she knew the names of several of the presidential candidates, but her knowledge was limited because "I really don't like to read much anymore, and CNN makes me nervous." Amelia's husband reported that Amelia was impatient about learning new information. Usually she asked him to operate their television remote control, even though they had had the same device for years. What really bothered him, though, was her disinterest in leaving their home and the amount of time she spent resting in bed. Most importantly, I learned from Amelia's husband that although her symptoms interfered with her life, they had not been becoming worse over the past few years.

I also reviewed Amelia's brain scans and ordered psychological testing. Her neurologist had ordered an EEG and CT scan of her brain. Both were unremarkable. Psychological testing did not show a significant compromise in her memory, and most of her skills were judged typical of women her age. Two rating scales revealed that she has ADHD, inattentive type.

This is not the presentation of a patient with dementia. In Alzheimer's disease, there is an inexorable decline in functioning, and Amelia's lack of progression was a good sign. Although her presentation was not consistent with dementia, it was not normal behavior. I informed Amelia that she had CFS. Although she and her husband were wary of this revised diagnosis, she agreed to add a long-acting stimulant to her medications.

Within a short time, it became clear that Amelia was responding well to treatment. She was gratified to find that the new medication tempered her brain fog. For the first time in years, Amelia was interested in reading the newspaper and finding books in the library. She no longer spent her days in bed and actually had the energy to take a trip with her husband. In my waiting room, she was holding a *Frommer's* travel guide with one hand and was writing notes with the other hand.

One does not hear many stories about patients who are pleased about a CFS diagnosis, but Amelia was one such person. Six months after treatment started, she told me, "I don't know if I am happier that my brain fog has improved or for knowing that I don't have Alzheimer's disease. For the past couple of years, I thought I was going to end up suffering like my mother-in-law. I am so relieved." The dread of living with an inaccurate diagnosis of dementia is quite cruel, and as I am certain that Amelia's odyssey is not unique, it is paramount for doctors to make a diagnosis of dementia accurately. A patient is placed in peril if CFS is dismissed from consideration of cognitive impairment.

Understanding "Cognition"

First, let's explore the concept of cognition. Cognition refers to the ability to think and reason clearly and includes the capacity to learn and remember new things. Many of us remain cognitively intact as we age, although there is some natural decline. As a rule, individuals in their 80s process information slower than they did in in their 50s. Compromised cognitive functioning can be displayed early in life and may be subtle at first. Children with ADHD and learning disabilities often misjudge time, forget names, and do not filter private thoughts.

Other circumstances can cause cognitive deficiencies. Young athletes are at risk for concussions resulting from contact sports. Concussive symptoms that include disorientation and confusion usually improve over time. Individuals who have repeated injuries may develop irreversible changes to their brains and behavior, a condition known as chronic traumatic encephalopathy (CTE). Cognitive changes increase with age. Dementia connotes a steadily declining mental ability, and there are many causes and phases of the condition. Patients with dementia have impaired memory and lack mental sharpness; as the disease progresses, they may neglect basic grooming and demonstrate poor social judgment.

In this book I argue that ADHD, chronic pain syndromes, and CFS (or combinations of these conditions) can explain many cases of more mild cognitive impairment. This is not widely known in the medical community; often CFS is overlooked, and struggling patients are given an inaccurate, albeit more established, diagnosis associated with cognitive impairment. The following conditions have been well described and represent various types of brain disease. Common to them all is that they are often confused with CFS, and they all lack good treatment. In contrast, brain fog associated with CFS has an effective treatment in the form of long-acting psychostimulants. For this reason, doctors must consider CFS as they sort out the diagnosis behind cognitive complaints.

Alzheimer's Disease (AD)

Alzheimer's disease is the most common form of dementia. Alzheimer's disease constitutes about 60 percent of cases of dementia, representing about six million people in the United States.[5] This illness was first described by Alois Alzheimer in 1906, and although diseases are no longer named for people, Dr. Alzheimer was immortalized by his finding. More than a hundred years later, there are still no practical blood tests or brain scans that can detect the presence of Alzheimer's disease in a living person, so the illness is diagnosed by symptoms. The earliest clue is nighttime confusion; the symptoms progress from there. Patients with advanced Alzheimer's disease require total care by others.

The exact cause of Alzheimer's disease is unknown, but it may be related to the clumps of a protein substance known as amyloid that have been found in the brains of deceased people with Alzheimer's disease. There is a genetic component, and a minority of people whose parents had Alzheimer's are at increased risk for developing the disease themselves.

Early-onset Alzheimer's disease refers to people with this disease whose symptoms occur before age 65; many people with this form of Alzheimer's are in their forties or fifties. Only about 200,000 people in the United States have early-onset Alzheimer's disease.[6] As with all others with Alzheimer's disease, their symptoms inexorably worsen over time. The medications for Alzheimer's disease are most effective when used in the early or moderate stages of the illness and at best delay the progression of the disease for a few years. There is no cure for any form of Alzheimer's disease, and nothing of significant promise is lurking on the horizon.

The common symptoms of Alzheimer's disease include some or all the following:

- Confusion over where the person is
- Confusion over what year it is
- Frequently losing items in odd places, such as putting socks in the refrigerator
- Difficulty with speaking or writing
- Using poor judgment, such as giving money or other items to others who may prey on them

There are five medications that are approved by the FDA for the treatment of Alzheimer's disease as of this writing, including rivastigmine (Exelon), galantamine (Razadyne), donepezil (Aricept), memantine (Namenda), and memantine combined with donepezil (Namzaric). Unfortunately, none of these medications reverses the symptoms of dementia; rather, they delay the rate of inevitable decline.

Vascular Dementia

Vascular dementia is the second most common form of dementia. It is present in up to 30 percent of all cases of dementia,[7] and it causes symptoms of brain fog similar to Alzheimer's disease. High blood pressure and damage to the circulatory system after a stroke can cause blockage or reduction of the blood flow to the brain, resulting in tissue damage. In the presence of cognitive impairment, brain scans may distinguish vascular dementia from Alzheimer's disease.

With vascular dementia, the symptoms are most likely to be difficulty with judgment and making decisions, and the person may have problems with balance and gait (walking). Some people have both vascular dementia and Alzheimer's disease.[8]

No medications have been approved specifically to treat vascular dementia, but these patients may be treated with the same medications approved for Alzheimer's disease. As with Alzheimer's, the benefits of these medication are modest.

Mild Cognitive Impairment (MCI)

Mild cognitive impairment includes some of the symptoms of Alzheimer's disease or vascular dementia (such as losing items or forgetting names), but it does not rise to the level of severity of even the first stages of dementia. According to the National Institute on Aging (NIA), symptoms of MCI may include forgetting appointments or events, frequently losing items, and having greater difficulty than nonimpaired people of the same age.[9]

The diagnosis of MCI often emerges when the doctor learns that his patient may have experienced a head injury or concussion at some time in the past and concludes that the patient's current complaints are the result of the head trauma. Since X-rays or other types of brain scans may or may not confirm such an injury, MCI is more of a description than a specific diagnosis. Some people with MCI may stay the same or return to normal functioning. Other patients with apparent MCI experience a worsening of their symptoms until a diagnosis of Alzheimer's disease or another form of dementia becomes apparent. According to the Alzheimer's Association, up to 20 percent of people aged 65 years and older may have MCI from any cause.[10]

Sometimes MCI is caused by a vitamin deficiency such as a deficiency in vitamin B12,[11] and before anyone is diagnosed with MCI, they should be tested for vitamin deficiencies. Major depression can also cause an impairment in thinking and should be ruled out before MCI is considered. Both vitamin deficiencies and depression account for some cases of MCI and are highly treatable conditions.

Chronic Traumatic Encephalopathy (CTE)

First diagnosed in boxers who were repeatedly hit in the head and were called "punch drunk," CTE is a disorder of individuals who have taken major blows to the head, causing brain trauma. Athletes may be subject to CTE, such as football players, hockey players, and soccer players. Military members exposed to explosions or combat conditions are also at risk for CTE, as are victims of head trauma sustained during domestic abuse.

People with CTE have cognitive impairment and may exhibit impulsive behavior, substance misuse, suicidal thoughts, and emotional instability. These symptoms may develop directly after a head injury or even years later. CTE is difficult to diagnose and not well understood.[12] This problem may be treated with CBT to help individuals cope with mood changes, memory training exercises to improve memory deficits, and massage or medications for individuals with recurrent headaches.[13] See Table 9.1 for a comparison of the brain fog of CFS to the brain confusion of chronic brain diseases.

Stimulant Medications Help

Clearly, CFS must be distinguished from other neurological conditions as it has a much different prognosis and more hopeful treatments. Long-acting stimulant medications, while currently not FDA approved for CFS, are at the center of this hope.

I have discussed the use of stimulants in earlier parts of the book. Chapter 5 describes the Rochester Study, which compared the long-acting stimulant LDX (Vyvanse) to placebo in 26 adult subjects with CFS. The study was designed to compare how the two groups fared with regard to fatigue, anxiety, and pain, and in each of these domains, the group treated with LDX outperformed the placebo group. The primary outcome measure of the Rochester Study was the BRIEFA, a neuropsychological assessment that closely captures the symptoms of brain fog. Overall, the group treated with LDX improved significantly more than the placebo-treated group. BRIEFA can be broken down to 10 subtasks; the test has the capacity to measure how well subjects can plan, organize, self-monitor, and shift their attention. In each of these subtests, LDX did better than placebo. The Rochester Study also demonstrated that LDX is well tolerated and has other benefits. If the study results hold up when it is replicated, there is hope that CFS patients suffering from brain fog will find relief with carefully monitored use of long-acting stimulant medication.

Table 9.1 Comparing Brain Fog in CFS and Chronic Brain Diseases

	Diagnosed with Brain Imaging Scans?	Caused by Head Injury?	Medications Help?	Prognosis?
Chronic fatigue syndrome	No	No	Yes	Improves with treatment, although not cured.
Vascular dementia	Yes	No	Medications that lower blood pressure reduce the chances or further damage due to stroke. Current medications do not reverse cognitive impairment.	Condition may worsen if strokes continue.
Early Alzheimer's disease	No (can be diagnosed after death by examining brain tissue)	No	Mildly, medications reduce rate of cognitive decline in early AD.	Condition always worsens
Mild cognitive impairment	No	Sometimes. MCI can result from concussion.	No, unless the person is deficient in vitamins, especially B12. If deficiency is corrected, condition will improve. Other types of MCI do not improve,	If caused by vitamin deficiency, it may be reversible. Sometimes progresses to dementia.
Chronic traumatic encephalopathy	Sometimes	Yes	No	Condition may worsen

Sources: Alzheimer's Association, "A Public Health Approach to Alzheimer's and Other Dementias: Module 2: Alzheimer's and Other Dementias—The Basics," https://www.cdc.gov/aging/aginginfo/pdfs/A-Public-Health-Approach-To-Alzheimers.pdf (accessed June 20, 2019); National Institute on Aging, "What Is Mild Cognitive Impairment?" May 16, 2017, https://www.nia.nih.gov/health/what-mild-cognitive-impairment (accessed June 21, 2019); Mayo Clinic, "Chronic Traumatic Encephalopathy," June 4, 2019, https://www.mayoclinic.org/diseases-conditions/chronic-traumatic-encephalopathy/symptoms-causes/syc-20370921 (accessed June 20, 2019); Concussion Legacy Foundation, "What Is CTE?" n.d., https://concussionfoundation.org/CTE-resources/what-is-CTE (accessed June 20, 2019).

Decluttering Her Home Helped Her Brain Fog

"One thing that really helped me was decluttering my house. It was too hard for me to start the project, so I actually hired a professional organizer to help me at first, and she trained me how to maintain an uncluttered life. After a couple weeks working together, my trash filled half the driveway. Then I gave away furniture that we were never going to use and old clothes that were not coming back in style. I would clean out a pile of collected treasures, post a free ad, and people would come and take the items. I belong to a Buy Nothing group, and anytime someone posts a need and I have it, then away goes the item. The house has much less clutter now, and I spend way less time cleaning it than in the past, which means much less stress for me. When you have brain fog, the more that you can reduce your personal stress levels, the better your life is. Decluttering is what worked for me."

Other Techniques to Resolve Brain Fog

Stimulants will play an important role in treatment, but they are not the only way to resolve brain fog. Below are some key ways to improve your brain fog problem:

- Exercise your body
- Exercise your brain
- Stop trying to multitask everything
- Make lists
- Keep your car keys in the same place, always
- Minimize stress
- Make time for friends and fun
- Find something to laugh about

Exercise Your Body

Physical exercise is an important elixir for most people with chronic fatigue and brain fog. It may seem like a paradox, but one of the most effective ways to counteract fatigue is with physical exertion. Exercise unleashes a torrent of chemicals in the brain that serve to improve cognitive functioning. I am struck by the number of people in my practice whose fatigue and cognitive complaints peaked after a minor orthopedic injury. At first, I thought these patients were reacting negatively to the pain of the injury or maybe the inconvenience of needing to use crutches for a few weeks. Instead, I realized that their symptoms were worse because they had abruptly stopped exercise. The biochemical bonanza of daily exercise that enhanced their cognition was suddenly gone, and the injury tipped their symptoms into more severe territory. Assertive efforts to rehabilitate quickly from injury are essential. It is wise to be creative and flexible. If a broken tibia prevents you from running, transition into upper body exercise. Just don't stop moving.

Exercise Your Brain

In a minority of patients with CFS, vigorous physical exercise will wear them out, and overexertion intensifies the fatigue. But it is always a good idea is to exercise your brain. Rediscover brainteaser activities that you once liked, such as crossword puzzles or Sudoku. Dust off your old Rubik's cylinder (harder than a Rubik's cube). Learn new video games; mastering virtual reality games will help stimulate your brain and condition you for more practical tasks of everyday life. The brain is a muscle—use it.

Stop Excessive Multitasking

The digital world has pushed people to perform multitasking to unsustainable levels and complicates efforts to overcome brain fog. Conducting business on the phone while driving in rush-hour traffic and admonishing a child in the back seat to stop kicking his brother is exhausting and often injurious to the person suffering from brain fog.

In these demanding situations, it's best to slow things down. Pay attention to the traffic now and talk to your children or your business associates later. Limit the noise in car—the radio need not be playing and competing with the children's video games. As experienced parents know, children usually exceed our expectations. Unless one child is likely to maul other child, they can probably manage for the short drive without your direct intervention.

Consider Meditation

"Meditation has helped me the most. It calms me and helps me to think more clearly. Instead of agonizing over how bad I feel or what I am supposed to be doing that I can't do because I feel so tired and sick, meditation makes me feel at peace. Meditation helps calm my worries, relaxes my body, and helps me feel more focused on what is most important in my life."

Incorporating meditation into your routine can be very simple, and you need not radically change your lifestyle or core beliefs. Melissa Oleshansky, PhD, is a clinical health psychologist and certified yoga instructor who incorporates mindfulness into her work with CFS patients. She offers some basic meditation techniques.

Find a place where you can be alone and without interruption. Relax the body in a comfortable seated position. Soften your shoulders. Gently close your eyes as a way to minimize external distraction. Bring awareness to your breath.

Breathe in slowly and deeply through the nose. Then gently open the lips, and slowly let all the air out. Pay attention to only your breathing. Breathe in again. Slowly let the breath out. This breath is longer than the natural breath. Try counting in your head to the number four on the in breath. Pause. Exhale out for a count of four. Continue with this rhythmic breath.

If the mind gets distracted, observe the thought, breathe in deeply, and then let go of the thought with your exhale. Free your mind of thoughts with your deep breathing meditation.

Practice this for a few minutes. Don't put a time limit on your meditation, or you may find yourself anxiously watching the clock for when you are supposed to stop, defeating a major part of the purpose of this exercise, which is to focus on your breathing as a way to relax the mind and the body. Dr. Oleshansky asserts that people with CFS are prone to taking shallow, rapid breaths rather than slow, deep breaths. Regular meditation will help patients with CFS get into the rhythm of breathing more normally and more healthfully while feeling an overall sense of peace and calm.

When you feel you are finished meditating, then you *are* finished. Practice the techniques daily—once in the morning and once in the evening, if possible. This practice, coupled with other techniques discussed above, will enhance mental and physical health.

Make Lists and Keep Them in a Central Place

Another way to combat brain fog is to give yourself reminders of appointments and major events. Buy a daily calendar with one page for each day, and as soon as you arrive home, staple the appointment card to the appropriate page. Similarly, put appointments directly into your phone applications—never wait until later to add new information. Also mark when important events will occur, such as family members' birthdays and major holidays (don't assume you would never forget them—it happens.) Break down a task into its elements and then create a to-do checklist. Keep the list on your phone or on a clipboard next to your bed. Don't forget; if you lose your routine, you will lose valuable time and exacerbate your fatigue.

Keep Important Items in the Same Place

Whether it's your car/house keys, your wallet/purse, your cell phone, or other items that you need nearly every day, make sure these items have their own "home" in your home or workplace. For example, when you arrive home from work, create a place where your items "live," and stick to it. So many people arrive home from work and drop their belongings wherever they are standing, and that can be a disaster in the making for a person with cognitive issues.

Minimize Stress as Much as Possible

Concentrate on your own problems and issues, and whenever possible, try to de-emphasize even these stressors. Also, choose your worry battles. Many people worry about problems that their children, including adult children, are experiencing, and they may even lose sleep worrying about the problems of other people. Decide which problems are yours to own. Here's one way to decide if you own a problem. Can you solve the problem by your own actions, or does someone else need to do something to solve the problem? If you can't change or influence someone else, or solve an issue by your own actions, then it is not your problem. We all have many problems, certainly enough to occupy our thoughts. So don't go out and adopt the problems of your family members and friends.

Make Some Time for Friends and Fun

It's important to not shut out the people in your life who matter to you. You may feel like they don't want to see you looking miserable, and of course true friends don't want you to be unhappy and sick. But they also care about you as an individual, so try to stay in contact with the major people in your life, whether a parent, a special aunt or cousin, or a close friend. Even a text or an occasional e-mail can keep you in each other's personal radar.

Laughter: Maybe the Best Medicine

There are times for everyone when life is harrowing and stressful, but when you get the chance to laugh aloud, take it! Better yet, generate opportunities for yourself, whether you love reading puns that others groan about or you like witty jokes or silly jokes that others don't appreciate at all.

Pacing Herself Helped

"I think dealing with this illness is all about pacing yourself. I used to have difficulty talking on the phone, and I couldn't read a book for several years. Now I can do both with ease, although I need to be careful to limit the length and frequency of each task. I've learned what and how much I can do now, and I don't fight my personal limits. Instead, I work with it. It's a much better way to live."

Do's and Don'ts Regarding Your Brain Fog

I have included some basic do's and don'ts to serve as daily guidance about how to, and how not to, approach brain fog:

- Don't panic
- Don't blame yourself
- Do ask for help from others
- Do be optimistic

Don't Panic

Freaking out about your brain fog will not resolve this problem—and it may make it worse. Getting upset because you can't remember where you put your cell phone or you forgot what time your appointment is will not help you recall the information that you are missing. Instead, when you have CFS, slow and steady wins the race. Take deep breaths and give yourself a break and a chance to regroup and rethink your situation.

Don't Blame Yourself

This brain fog problem is not your fault—really! So stop condemning yourself to others and in your own mind. You're not stupid, and you're not a bad person. People with CFS frequently have executive dysfunction; it's part of the entire syndrome, just like the fatigue and the pain. This is unfortunate, but it's true. You are at fault no more than people who struggle with other medical challenges.

You don't expect a person in a wheelchair to suddenly leap out of the chair and bound down the street. And neither should you expect a person with brain fog from chronic CFS to rapidly overcome her executive skills issues. It's not your fault. That is worth saying one more time!

Do Ask for Help from Others

When you are having a problem with thinking, sometimes it helps to ask others for assistance. "My husband and my daughter are my rocks," said Arlene. "When I struggle to locate missing items, and no matter how hard I try, I can't find them, I ask them to help me. And they always do! They ask me questions about when I had the item last, where I was when I had it, and so on, and together we nearly always solve the problem. You don't have to do everything on your own, all the time."

Do Be Optimistic

If you have often or always been a "glass half-empty" kind of person who tends to look askance at whatever happens to you, that needs to change. Like a man dying of thirst in the desert who turns up his nose at a gift of water that's a little murky, this strategy won't work well for you. Work to accentuate the positive. Try to avoid forecasting predictions of a bad outcome. Statements like "This treatment won't help me because nothing ever does" epitomize this unproductive type of self-talk.

But if your mood remains down, and the bulk of your thoughts are pessimistic, you and your doctor might consider an antidepressant medication. Brain fog and CFS constitute a huge burden made harder if you always feel negative. Cognitive Behavioral Therapy and antidepressant medication can play an important role in improving your outlook.

This chapter was all about brain fog and ways to improve it, but there's still one important subject left to cover, and that is sleep. Chapter 10 is all about sleep issues that many people with chronic fatigue experience, whether it's insomnia, restless legs, or other sleep problems—and it's also about how to resolve these issues.

Notes

1. Karen B. Schmaling and Betterton, Karran L., "Neurocognitive Complaints and Functional Status among Patients with Chronic Fatigue Syndrome and Fibromyalgia," *Quality Life Research* 25, n. 5 (May 2016): 1257–1263.

2. Ibid.

3. Anthony J. Ocon, "Caught in the Thickness of Brain Fog: Exploring the Cognitive Symptoms of Chronic Fatigue Syndrome," *Frontiers in Physiology* 4, n. 63 (April 2013), https://www.ncbi.nlm.nih.gov/pmc /articles/PMC3617392/pdf/fphys-04-00063.pdf (accessed May 22, 2019).

4. Ibid.

5. Alzheimer's Association, *2019 Alzheimer's Disease Facts and Figures*. Chicago, IL: Alzheimer's Association, 2019. https://www.alz.org /media/Documents/alzheimers-facts-and-figures-2019-r.pdf (accessed June 20, 2019).

6. Alzheimer's Association, "A Public Health Approach to Alzheimer's and Other Dementias: Module 2: Alzheimer's and Other Dementias—The Basics," https://www.cdc.gov/aging/aginginfo/pdfs/A -Public-Health-Approach-To-Alzheimers.pdf (accessed June 20, 2019).

7. Ibid.

8. Alzheimer's Association, *2019 Alzheimer's Disease Facts and Figures*. Chicago, IL: Alzheimer's Association, 2019. https://www.alz.org /media/Documents/alzheimers-facts-and-figures-2019-r.pdf (accessed June 20, 2019).

9. National Institute on Aging, "What Is Mild Cognitive Impairment?" May 16, 2017, https://www.nia.nih.gov/health/what-mild-cognitive -impairment (accessed June 21, 2019).

10. Ibid.

11. Alzheimer's Association, "A Public Health Approach to Alzheimer's and Other Dementias: Module 2: Alzheimer's and Other Dementias—The Basics," https://www.cdc.gov/aging/aginginfo/pdfs/A -Public-Health-Approach-To-Alzheimers.pdf (accessed June 20, 2019).

12. Mayo Clinic, "Chronic Traumatic Encephalopathy," June 4, 2019, https://www.mayoclinic.org/diseases-conditions/chronic-traumatic -encephalopathy/symptoms-causes/syc-20370921 (accessed June 20, 2019).

13. Concussion Legacy Foundation, "What Is CTE?" n.d., https:// concussionfoundation.org/CTE-resources/what-is-CTE (accessed June 20, 2019).

CHAPTER 10

Sleep: Why It's Important and How to Get Enough

" *I've been diagnosed with chronic fatigue syndrome, and it seems accurate because I have fatigue, chronic pain, and brain fog. So how in the world can it be that I'm exhausted throughout the day, but I lie awake practically every night? I just don't understand this, and it's making me crazy. Is insomnia normal in a person with my problem? And is it even treatable? Does anyone else with chronic fatigue ever have this problem—and if they do, what can they do about it?" asked a very frustrated Miranda.*

Sleep is crucially important to everyone's good health, but getting a good night's sleep is a common problem experienced by many people with CFS. This chapter explores chronic insomnia, sleep apnea, and restless legs syndrome (RLS) and offers ideas on how to address these key sleep issues. Most research studies have shown that when chronic insomnia is treated, other problems areas such as pain and fatigue also improve.[1]

Sleep is a concern for many adults; the CDC reports that more than a third of Americans (35%) don't get enough sleep.[2] Sleep problems are amplified among people with CFS when compared to other chronic neurological illness. Researchers compared sleep quality in patients with CFS and multiple sclerosis (MS) and found that 55 percent of the subjects with CFS reported severe, unrefreshed sleep. Among the patients with MS, 28 percent reported having this problem.[3]

In this chapter, I outline the common sleep disorders and the respective treatment that people with CFS confront. Nonpharmacological solutions such as improving sleep hygiene and incorporating stress-reducing techniques, such as progressive muscle relaxation, are explored. Many people are drawn to over-the-counter herbs and supplements such as chamomile or melatonin, and I describe the potential utility for these herbs and supplements. A word of caution: even though these drugs are "natural," they have some concerning side effects that should be understood.

Sometimes these approaches are not sufficient, and more decisive measures need to be taken. I describe prescription sleep medications and provide a discussion about what role each drug may play for patients with CFS.

The sleep disturbances so common to patients with CFS is rarely an isolated symptom; typically, other symptoms coexist and complicate the clinical presentation. For those who have chronic pain associated with insomnia, refer to the narrative and case studies in Chapter 8. In addition, many people with CFS suffer from problems with depression and anxiety, issues that are addressed in Chapter 4. This chapter also addresses medical conditions that may accompany or need to be distinguished from CFS.

Considering Insomnia

Insomnia has many component parts. The most common definition is the inability to sleep, usually a problem for people who need to sleep at night. But there are other aspects of insomnia, such as having trouble falling asleep, frequent awakenings, having trouble getting back to sleep once you have woken up, and feeling unrefreshed from sleep when you eventually do wake up—no matter how many hours you have slept. Insufficient or nonrestorative sleep at night may lead to excessive daytime sleepiness. Insomnia is linked to numerous problems, such as trouble concentrating, memory problems, and an overall reduced quality of life.[4]

In general, women are more likely to suffer from insomnia than men, and not everyone shares the same risk for developing the sleep disturbance. Specific insomnia risks include having an irregular work schedule (midnight nurses have high rates of sleep disruption) or having sleep apnea or fibromyalgia. Individuals experiencing high levels of psychological stress, recurrent depression, or other mental health problems are also at risk.[5]

Most people with CFS complain about daytime fatigue and the general assumption, advanced by research included later in the next section, is that improved nighttime sleep remedies daytime fatigue. That is not always true. Nighttime sleep integrity is essential, but it does not ensure a sense of well-being in the daytime. In other words, for many individuals with CFS, treatment with morning medications, specifically long-acting stimulants, remains necessary even in the presence of ideal nighttime sleep. For a fuller discussion of treatment for daytime fatigue, refer to Chapters 5 and 6.

Resolving Your Insomnia May Decrease Daytime Fatigue

Programs that address psychosocial and insomnia difficulties of CFS patients reveal that participants reported less daytime fatigue. Norwegian researchers assembled 122 subjects with chronic fatigue syndrome and provided a 3.5-week comprehensive course of rehabilitation and return-to-work therapy. The researchers found that by addressing their insomnia, the subjects enjoyed a significant improvement in their fatigue as well as in their ability to recover from stressful situations. The researchers concluded, "Insomnia severity may be a maintaining factor in chronic fatigue and specifically targeting this in treatment could increase treatment response."[1]

Note

1. Havard Kallestad, et al., "The Role of Insomnia in the Treatment of Chronic Fatigue," *Journal of Psychosomatic Research* 78 (2015): 1.

Do You Have Good Sleep Hygiene?

People practice good hygiene in other daily routines, such as washing their hands before preparing food, brushing their teeth after meals (or at least once a day), and taking showers. Here are some of the basics of good sleep hygiene that can significantly improve the life of a person with insomnia:

- Use your bedroom for sleep and sex only
- Go to bed at the same time every night
- Stop worrying about not sleeping
- Avoid clock watching
- Avoid caffeine (chocolate, coffee, or tea) after dinner
- Could it be your medication?
- No alcohol before bed
- No big meals before bedtime

Use Your Bedroom for Sleep and Sex Only

People struggling with insomnia should limit the scope of their bedroom's function. Some people decide bedtime is a great time to read e-mails, send texts, or rage on Twitter. Very bad idea! All these activities and even something as noninteractive as reading are stimulating and are known to hinder active sleep.

Nor is your bedroom a good place to perform your daily exercises—keep that health living activity in the gym. Instead, limit your bedroom to two functions: sleep and sex. If you get into the mind-set that these two activities are the purpose of your bedroom, then you are less likely to fall into the unconscious habit of thinking that you need your television, tablet, or other devices to entertain you. One more thing: no snacking in your bedroom at any time.

Go to Bed at the Same Time Every Night

The brain craves repetition, and one essential routine for good sleep is to go to sleep at the same time every night. More importantly, it is important to wake up at approximately the same time every morning. You may deserve to stay up later weekends and holidays; unlimited sleeping in is a core pleasure for many people. That might be acceptable choice for a person who does not have insomnia problem, but for those who do have insomnia, waking up at noon on Saturday and Sunday will make the 7:00 a.m. alarm on Monday morning very disruptive.

Stop Worrying about Not Sleeping

Most of us have found ourselves awake at midnight or 1:00 a.m., when we know that we must wake up at 7:00 a.m. to get ready for work. So what do we do? We worry that we only have *six more hours* to sleep. So hurry up brain. Get to sleep. Then it's 2:00 a.m. and 3:00 a.m., and as the clock ticks, it is easy to get panic-stricken about the limited amount of time that's left. Does this type of thinking help a person relax into Dreamland? It does not! Excessive worry has the opposite effect. Have faith that your body will regulate itself and will adjust to occasional exposure to short sleep nights.

Avoid Clock Watching

You may need an alarm clock to wake you up in time in the morning, but that does not mean the face of the clock needs to be visible to you.

Simply get up, shut the alarm off, and start your day. Clock watching is like panicking as the time passes, but it requires a clock. Turn it around so you cannot see it. It will still go off at the right time in the morning. If you normally wear a watch in the daytime, take it off at night and put it face down and out of reach.

Generally, Stay Away from Caffeine after Dinner

Caffeine is a stimulant, which is why substances containing caffeine should be avoided after the later afternoon. Coffee, tea, coffee, and many carbonated soft drinks have high caffeine content and are associated with excitation of the nervous system. Every once in a while, however, the opposite is true. I have a few patients who report that caffeine allows them to relax and focus on falling asleep. So while staying stimulant free is generally advised, there are exceptions to the rule.

Avoid Daytime Naps

You may think naps must be healthy, because don't people in other countries take regular siestas? That may be part of their culture, but unless it is also part of yours, afternoon naps—or any naps—are a bad idea. Naps will train your body to need fewer hours of nighttime sleep. In addition, regular naps will worsen insomnia. In well-run nursing homes, the elderly are purposely kept busy during the day to discourage napping and to promote nighttime sleep patterns.

Could the Problem with Insomnia Be Related to Your Medications?

Some medications, including some over-the-counter medicines, may cause delay sleep onset. Certain over-the-counter cold and flu medications can prevent or delay sleep because they contain caffeine or phenylephrine. Pseudoephedrine, a more potent decongestant, is more highly regulated in select states and dramatically impairs sleep. Other medications may have an activating effect, including the stimulants that I discus extensively in other chapters for counteracting the effects of chronic fatigue. There are times when stimulant medication needs to be given in the afternoon (generally to augment waning doses given in the morning), but the effects on sleep need to carefully considered before afternoon dosing is undertaken. Other commonly used medications that may cause insomnia include beta-blockers, clonidine, and antidepressants that block the reuptake of serotonin such as fluoxetine (Prozac).

No Alcohol before Bed

A few shots of alcohol before bedtime has been suggested, but this is not a sustainable practice over time. What usually happens is the person falls asleep (or passes out) in the evening and then wake up hours later, dehydrated and with throbbing head pain. The effect on next day functioning are not good. Binge drinking is not a desirable way to restore basic sleep needs, but a glass of wine may be helpful on occasion.

No Big Meals before Bedtime

It may be Parisian to eat a sumptuously large meal at 8:00 p.m. or 9:00 p.m. or later, but when you plan to go to bed at 11:00 p.m., the heavy load of food may make proper digestion pretty challenging. In many households, the "big meal of the day" is the evening meal, but it might be prudent to consume dense calories earlier in the day. Certainly, a large noon meal may also cause a person to get sleepy. Think how soporific the midday Thanksgiving meal is, when many people gorge themselves, and afterward, all they want to do is lie down and sleep.

Herbal or Supplemental Remedies

Sometimes people with sleep problems don't want to take prescribed medications, but they know they need extra help to overcome their insomnia. In such cases, sleep problems may be improved by taking melatonin or herbal remedies like chamomile, valerian, kava, or passionflower. (Some of these come in the form of teas.) Keep in mind that all drugs come with both benefits and side effects, and alternative remedies derived from natural plants are no exception to this rule; for example, cobra venom and opium are natural substances, but it's best to stay clear of them. See Table 10.1 for a listing of possible supplements that may help you obtain the sleep you need.

Some herbs and supplements interact with other medications, which means that they may increase, decrease, or completely counteract the effects of other drugs that you may take. For example, in the past, sometimes St. John's Wort was used for depression and for insomnia; however, this herb causes so many dangerous interactions with multiple drugs that it generally should be avoided. For example, it can stop birth control pills from working, increase the effect of a blood thinner, and reverse the effects of chemotherapy drugs taken by cancer patients—and these are only a few of the potentially problematic effects.

Table 10.1 Considering the Pros and Cons of Herbal/Supplemental Sleep Remedies

Name	Herb or Supplement?	Possible Side Effects and Warnings
Chamomile	Herb	Patients may be allergic to it, especially people allergic to ragweed, chrysanthemums, daisies, or marigolds; should not be used by people taking the blood thinner warfarin or cyclosporine, a drug used to prevent organ transplant rejections.
Melatonin	Supplement	May cause headaches, nausea, and dizziness.
Valerian	Herb	May cause headache, dizziness, digestive disturbances, and itching.
Kava	Herb	May harm the liver
Passionflower	Herb	Should not be used during pregnancy because it may induce contractions.
St. John's Wort	Herb	Interacts with many drugs, such as MAOI antidepressants, birth control pills, warfarin, some cancer medications. Side effects may include dry mouth, dizziness, headache, anxiety, sexual dysfunction.

Sources: National Center for Complementary and Integrative Health, "Chamomile," September 2016, https://nccih.nih.gov/health/chamomile/ataglance.htm (accessed June 10, 2019); Darren J. Hein, "OTC Insomnia Supplements: The Latest Evidence" March 15, 2019, https://www.medscape.com/viewarticle/910144_3 (accessed June 10, 2019); National Center for Complementary and Integrative Health, "Valerian," September 2016, https://www.medscape.com/viewarticle/910144_3 (accessed June 12, 2019); National Center for Complementary and Integrative Health, "Melatonin: In Depth," May 2015, https://nccih.nih.gov/health/melatonin (accessed June 10, 2019); National Center for Complementary and Integrative Health, "Passionflower," September 2016, https://nccih.nih.gov/health/passionflower (accessed June 10, 2019).

Be sure to tell your physician before trying any herbs or supplements to help with resolving a problem with insomnia. Bear in mind that many health care providers are not familiar with the intricacies of supplements for several reasons. First, the FDA does not consider these supplements medications, so they are not subjected to the same rigorous scientific testing as prescribed medications. Usually there is no existing data exploring long-term safety, and the impact the supplement has on other medications is unknown. Second, the quality control of food additives is not consistent. Some agents are imported from nations with lower drug purity standards. With supplements, the old mantra "Let the buyer beware" applies.

Sleep Medications for Chronic Insomnia

Sometimes prescribed sleep medications are needed to obtain sufficient sleep. Many people are apprehensive about taking sleep medications to treat their chronic insomnia, as they may be fearful of becoming dependent or have concerns that they might oversleep the next morning. In reality these medications are quite safe, assuming the user follows the physician's recommendations. Avoid alcohol and other drugs, especially opioids, when taking these sedative hypnotics.

Considering Specific Sleep Medications

The medications used most often for sleep are related to the benzodiazepine class. Some of the older antidepressants are also for sleep induction, albeit at lower doses than are used to elevate mood. Table 10.2 covers the most commonly prescribed sleep medications and discusses what type of medication each is, its key benefits, and common side effects that may occur with their use.

The benzodiazepine receptor agonist (BzRA) is a common category of sleep medications, and it includes such drugs as zaleplon (Sonata), Eszopiclone (Lunesta), and zolpidem (Ambien). These drugs are specifically approved by the FDA for treating insomnia, and their pharmacological effects are more directed on sleep than benzodiazepines like alprazolam (Xanax) and diazepam (Valium). Melatonin is a readily available sleep remedy that engages natural melatonin receptors in the body to induce sedation and sleep. The melatonin receptor agonist drug ramelteon (Rozerem) also exploits the melatonin pathways. The orexin receptor antagonist suvorexant (Belsomra) is a newer category of sleep medication; it reverses the natural wakefulness of the orexin/hypocretin system in the body.[6]

An older but often overlooked antidepressant, doxepin (Silenor), is specifically approved by the FDA as a treatment for chronic insomnia. Trazadone (Desyrel) is also an antidepressant, and though it never

Table 10.2 FDA-Approved Sleep Medications

Brand (Generic) Name	Type of Medication	Possible Side Effects
Zolpidem (Ambien, Ambien CR, Edluar, Intermezzo, and Zolpimist)	Benzodiazepine receptor agonist, also known as a non-benzodiazepine hypnotic	Headaches, sleepiness, falls
Esziopiclone (Lunesta)	Benzodiazepine receptor agonist	Metallic taste in the mouth, dizziness, headache, sleepiness
Zaleplon (Sonata)	Benzodiazepine receptor agonist	Drowsiness, headache, nausea, may worsen symptoms of depression in people with depressive disorders
Ramelton (Rozerem)	Melatonin Receptor Agonist	Sleepiness, dizziness, and fatigue
Suvorexant (Belsomra)	Orexin receptor agonist	Not recommended for patients with narcolepsy
Doxepin (Silenor)	Antidepressant	Drowsiness, dizziness, difficulty with urination, constipation, nausea and vomiting

Sources: Pradeep C. Ballu and Kaur, Harleen, "Sleep Medicine: Insomnia and Sleep," *Missouri Medicine* 116, n. 1 (January/February 2019): 68–75; John M. Eisenberg Center for Clinical Decisions and Communications Science, "Managing Insomnia Disorder: A Review of the Research for Adults," August 2017, https://www.ncbi.nlm.nih.gov/books/NBK537838/ (accessed June 12, 2019).

received official FDA clearance, it is frequently used off-label as a sleep-inducing medication.

What about Marijuana and CBD?

Marijuana and CBD oil were covered in depth in Chapter 8, where possible remedies for chronic pain are discussed. Assuming such substances are legal in their state, some readers find that these remedies may alleviate their insomnia. The chapter also addresses concerns about marijuana and CBD oil. Refer to that chapter, and take these issues into account before deciding on cannabis.

Considering Cognitive Behavioral Therapy for Insomnia (CBT-I)

Researchers have shown that CBT for insomnia is highly effective and usually resolves insomnia symptoms in 8–10 sessions or fewer. A CBT therapist collects a thorough history of the patient's insomnia problem and then makes individualized suggestions. Sometimes the suggestions revolve around improving sleep hygiene through science-based psychoeducation that busts common myths and misconceptions about sleep, such as "I must get at least eight hours of sleep to function." Participants in CBT-I find relief in learning that 100 percent of deep sleep occurs within 5.5 hours of sleep, and studies show that daytime performance is adequately maintained. Research also indicates that six–seven hours of sleep is associated with the longest life expectancy.

The therapist identifies mistakes that are commonly made, such as lying in bed at night, thinking about all your most challenging problems, or what you should have said when the boss or another person made a nasty comment to you that really rankles. Repetitive negative thoughts that occur before bed, during nighttime waking, and in the morning are captured by the patient and then replaced by helpful and true facts about sleep. Patients are given tools to track their sleep habits using a weekly time log and instructed how to calculate their sleep efficiency, which is the total amount of sleep divided by total time spent in bed. The cognitive behavioral therapist will help determine your key sleep issues and individualize the therapy to help you resolve your insomnia.

A CBT therapist usually can resolve insomnia problem in 8–10 sessions or fewer. The therapist will ask many questions about the patient's insomnia problem and then make individualized suggestions. Sometimes the suggestions revolve around improving sleep hygiene, but the therapist can also identify other mistakes that are commonly made, such as lying in bed at night ruminating about the day's events. The cognitive behavioral therapist will help determine your key sleep issues and individualize the therapy to help you resolve your insomnia issues.

In a study reported in 2018 in Korea, the researchers provided CBT-I to 41 subjects with insomnia, most of whom also received sleep medications. The control group of 100 subjects received pharmacotherapy (sleep medications) only. At the conclusion of the study, the researchers found that the CBT-I reduced the need for sleep medications in the study group significantly compared to the control group, and the case closure rate was higher—meaning those subjects no longer needed therapy.[7]

Other Therapies That Improve Chronic Insomnia Problems:
Progressive Muscle Relaxation

Progressive muscle relaxation is another approach that may help you get yourself to sleep and overcome your problems with chronic insomnia, particularly when you are feeling anxious. Progressive muscle relaxation basically involves mentally tightening and then loosening muscles in your body, starting with your toes and slowly moving up to your head and neck. This form of relaxation therapy helps to alleviate tension and stress as you concentrate on the parts of your body and helping each group of muscles tense and then relax, in a graduated, stepwise fashion.

I've adapted the step-by-step instructions provided by the Veterans Administration to military veterans who are battling insomnia.[8] The exercise takes about 10 minutes to complete and hopefully sleep will greet you before the exercise is complete. If not, start again and allow your body to transition to peaceful sleep.

1. Find a quiet place to sit or lie down.
2. Close your eyes if you can. If this makes you uncomfortable, you can keep your eyes open during this exercise.
3. Take very slow, deep breaths by inhaling through your nose with your mouth closed. Do this to a count of four.
4. Repeat this breathing exercise four times. But if you start to feel dizzy, go back to your normal breathing pattern.
5. Start at your feet, and as you inhale, tighten these muscles and hold the tension briefly. Then, as you breathe out, let all the tension flow out, as if it were coming out with your exhaled breath. Feel the difference between the tension phase and the relaxation phase.
6. Press the balls of the feet into the floor and raise your heels, allowing the calf muscles to contract. Feel this tension in the calves. Then release, and observe the muscles relaxing. Have the tension and relaxation match your breath. Then tighten the knees and allow your legs to straighten. Feel the lightness in the front of the legs and notice the tension while inhaling a breath. Then release on the exhale, allowing the legs to bend and relax back onto the floor.
7. Continue this tightening and relaxing process as you move up through the body. Move to the stomach and then to the hands and arms.
8. Finish the exercise by tensing the muscles in the face, tightening the face, and then letting all the tension flow out with the exhaling breath.

9. Notice if you feel any areas of tension that remain in the body and work on tightening and relaxing those areas.
10. At the end of the exercise, relax. And hopefully, you may fall fast asleep.

Considering Yoga, Meditation, or Tai Chi

In addition to the recommendations already made in this chapter, many readers may benefit from taking classes in yoga, meditation, or tai chi. These Eastern practices have been employed for millennia to enhance relaxation and promote healthy living. As with progressive muscle relaxation, these practices encourage mind-body integration. Many cities offer these programs in private studios, local gyms, or community centers.

Considering Sleep Apnea

Sleep apnea is characterized by short periods of breathing cessation during sleep. Individuals with this medical condition stop breathing for short periods during sleep. The condition may be suspected because of loud snoring (usually reported by a spouse or partner) and reported apneic periods of gasping and choking during sleep. The frequency and severity of the apnea events is assessed during a formal sleep study conducted in a sleep laboratory. Sleep apnea is most accurately diagnosed by a sleep specialist who can provide specialized treatment.

The most common type of OSA condition is caused by excessive soft tissue in the back of the throat that blocks the passage of air.[9] When this obstruction result in frequent apneas, deep and restorative sleep is nearly impossible to achieve. Impaired nighttime sleep results in excessive daytime sleepiness, and OSA patients may also suffer from headaches, irritability, difficulty concentrating, anxiety, and depression. According to the American Sleep Apnea Association, an estimated 22 million Americans experience sleep apnea, and many of them have gone undiagnosed despite having long-standing sleep disturbances. No one primary complaint characterizes the patient with OSA. Some report sleeping too much, but many others say that they have a problem falling asleep at the beginning of the night.[10]

Sleep apnea is helped by using pillows and other devices that keep patients from sleeping on their backs. Certain oral appliances that keep the airway open during sleep may be helpful. If these measures don't work, the person may receive a CPAP device that delivers humidified room air through a mask during sleep. Although some OSA patients object to wearing a device during sleep, improvements in mask design have allowed patients to better tolerate the device.[11]

Restless Legs Syndrome (RLS)

Restless legs syndrome (RLS) is a disorder that sounds like its name: the sufferer has a compelling sensation to move about when lying down. The sensations of RLS can feel like an aching or a creeping feeling, and although it is primarily experienced in the legs, it may also occur in the arms or even the head or chest. These sensations may range from annoying all the way up to painful and most often start in the lower extremities but can be felt throughout the body. Restlessness becomes most apparent at night when there is quiet and few distractions. Often there is little available to palliate the symptoms; the patient will resort to calisthenics or hot showers to decrease the discomfort. Usually the restlessness returns quickly and there is no time to transition into sleep. RLS causes daytime sleepiness and extreme fatigue, making it difficult to perform many daytime tasks. RLS symptoms have often been reported in individuals who suffer from ADHD. The National Institute of Neurological Disorders and Stroke estimates that RLS can decrease work productivity by as much as 20 percent.[12]

RLS appears to be an inherited disorder affecting up to 10 percent of American population divided equally between men and women[13] and can be related to iron deficiency and the consumption of caffeine, alcohol, or nicotine. RLS can emerge during pregnancy and self-resolve after birth.

Treatment for RLS includes avoiding exacerbating substances, such as caffeinated foods and beverages, alcohol, and tobacco. People low in iron should receive iron supplementation, and a deficiency is easily detected in a blood test.

Antiseizure drugs are usually the medications of choice to treat RLS, particularly gabapentin enacarbil (Horizant), which is specifically indicated for treatment of RLS. Gabapentin (Neurontin) or pregabalin (Lyrica) may also be used, and in certain cases, dopamine agonists such as ropinorole (Requip) and pramipexole (Mirapex) are prescribed. Benzodiazepines may also be prescribed, including clonazepam (Klonopin) or lorazepam (Ativan). Benzodiazepines are sedating and allow the individual to experience restful sleep; however, this class of medication should be used with considerable care, as it is habit-forming. Never take more than the prescribed dosage ordered by the physician.

Chronic insomnia is a complicating factor in the lives of many patients with CFS. There are many causes of insomnia and many treatment responses, ranging from changes in behavior to the use of medications or physical devices. To the persistent individual who seeks answers, explanations and solutions are available.

Notes

1. Havard Kallestad, et al., "The Role of Insomnia in the Treatment of Chronic Fatigue," *Journal of Psychosomatic Research* 78 (2015): 427–432.

2. Centers for Disease Control and Prevention, "1 in 3 Adults Don't Get Enough Sleep," February 16, 2016, https://www.cdc.gov/media /releases/2016/p0215-enough-sleep.html (accessed June 16, 2019).

3. Vageesh Jain, et al., "Prevalence of and Risk Factors for Severe Cognitive and Sleep Symptoms in ME/CFS and MS," *BMC Neurology* 17 (2017), https://www.ncbi.nlm.nih.gov/pmc/articles/PMC5477754 /pdf/12883_2017_Article_896.pdf (accessed June 10, 2019).

4. Jasvinder Chandra, "Insomnia," *Medscape*, September 11, 2018, https://emedicine.medscape.com/article/1187829 (accessed June 12, 2019).

5. Office of Women's Health, "Insomnia," November 30, 2017, https://www.womenshealth.gov/a-z-topics/insomnia (accessed June 10, 2019).

6. Pradeep C. Ballu and Kaur, Harleen, "Sleep Medicine: Insomnia and Sleep," *Missouri Medicine* 116, n. 1 (January/February 2019): 68–75.

7. Kyung Mee Park, et al., "Cognitive Behavioral Therapy for Insomnia Reduces Hypnotic Prescriptions," *Psychiatry Investigation* (2017), https://www.ncbi.nlm.nih.gov/pmc/articles/PMC5976005/pdf/pi-2017 -11-20.pdf (accessed June 10, 2019).

8. Veterans Administration Employment Toolkit, "Relaxation Exercise: Progressive Muscle Relaxation," n.d., https://www.va.gov/vetsin workplace/docs/em_eap_exercise_PMR.asp (accessed June 10, 2019).

9. American Sleep Apnea Association, "A Very Short Course on Sleep Apnea," n.d., https://www.sleepapnea.org/learn/sleep-apnea-information -clinicians/ (accessed June 12, 2019).

10. Jasvinder Chandra, "Insomnia," *Medscape*, September 11, 2018, https://emedicine.medscape.com/article/1187829 (accessed June 12, 2019).

11. National Institute of Neurological Disorders and Stroke, "Restless Legs Syndrome Fact Sheet," May 2017, https://www.ninds.nih.gov/disorders/patient-caregiver-education/fact-sheets/restless-legs-syndrome-fact-sheet (accessed June 16, 2019).

12. Ibid.

13. National Institute of Neurological Disorders and Stroke, "Restless Legs Syndrome Fact Sheet," May 2017, https://www.ninds.nih.gov/disorders/patient-caregiver-education/fact-sheets/restless-legs-syndrome-fact-sheet (accessed June 16, 2019).

Conclusion

Reading a book about a medical problem is akin to taking an intellectual journey with the author. The ideas and descriptions may initially feel similar to driving through unfamiliar terrain, perhaps passing over some untraveled, bumpy, cobblestone roads. But after learning more about the subject, the reader starts experiencing some *Aha!* moments, gaining new views and insights, similar to the way a driver might notice an intriguing café or a park that warrants further exploration. Hopefully, the author navigates you steadily through any rough spots and onto a clear path of understanding and empathy for the inhabitants of this little town—in this case, people who are burdened with CFS and who need and want help. The reader could also be a physician who wants to help their patients with this problem. This book could be the help that they have been denied for far too long.

In this book, I have discussed the key symptoms of CFS and explained how CFS is similar to and different from other diagnoses. This vital process is called the differential diagnosis, and it is a key fact-finding mission to help determine whether a person has CFS or another medical condition.

I have also discussed my own research study using a stimulant medication to successfully improve the lives of subjects who were diagnosed with CFS. I followed that discussion with a chapter on stimulant medications that may help patients with CFS, including both the pros and cons of amphetamines, methylphenidate, and wakefulness medications such as modafinil. My last four chapters focused on the key problems experienced by virtually every person with CFS and offered practical advice to resolve these issues. Such problems include fatigue, chronic pain, brain fog, and sleep problems.

As we wind this book down to its conclusion, I hope my readers will feel that they have gained the knowledge they need to navigate CFS and arrive at the much-needed solutions. I also hope they feel that they now understand this distressing medical problem and are armed and ready with the information they need. In effect, I hope readers feel that they have truly reached their destination.

APPENDIXES

Appendix A: Ten Frequently Asked Questions and Answers about Chronic Fatigue Syndrome

1. Q: How many people have CFS?
   A: At least 2.5 million people in the United States, according to the CDC. Some experts believe the number is higher, but the CDC is the best estimate.

2. Q: Does CFS have other names?
   A: Yes. Some experts use the term myalgic encephalomyelitis/chronic fatigue disorder (ME/CFS). The newest name for the disorder as of this writing is systemic exertion intolerance disease (SEID).

3. Q: Does everyone with CFS have severe fatigue?
   A: The severity of the fatigue varies from one person to the next, and it even varies within the same person, who may have good days and other days that are not so good. Some people with CFS are bedbound while others can work part-time, although it is often difficult for them.

4. Q: Are women more prone to a CFS diagnosis than men are?
   A: Women do seem to have a greater percentage of CFS diagnoses than men, but some studies indicate as many as 40 percent of people with CFS may be male.

5. Q: Do some people with CFS have other mental health issues?
   A: Yes, many have issues with depression, anxiety, and other mental health problems. These problems may seem huge to the person affected by them, but they are all treatable.

6. Q: Why do some doctors seem to think CFS is a fake diagnosis?
   A: Some doctors don't understand that CFS is a real problem, in part because many doctors prefer to treat measurable illnesses. For example, if a person has high blood pressure and is given medication, then the blood pressure should drop to a lower level. In contrast, fatigue is not easily quantifiable.

7. Q: Do many people with CFS have trouble with pain as well as fatigue?
   A: Yes, many of them do, and sometimes treatment helps resolve pain as well as fatigue.

8. Q: What about cognitive problems that some people call brain fog? Is that a real issue in people with chronic fatigue syndrome?
   A: Yes, many people with CFS have difficulty with thinking and concentrating; however, treatment can help to improve this condition.

9. Q: You have used prescribed stimulants to treat patients with chronic fatigue syndrome? What are the effects of stimulants?
   A: Stimulants help improve the energy level of most people with chronic fatigue syndrome. It may also decrease the perception of pain, at least in part, because active people are less likely to ruminate about how badly they are feeling. For some patients, stimulants completely turn their lives around.

10. Q: Are prescribed stimulants safe? Is there a risk of becoming a drug abuser?
    A: Prescribed stimulants are safe when a person takes the medication as the doctor has prescribed and does not share medication with others. The people most likely to abuse prescribed stimulants are college students, followed by young adults who are not college students. People in their late 20s and older rarely abuse prescribed stimulants, as I discuss in Chapter 6.

Appendix B: Glossary

This appendix includes words that may be unfamiliar to readers, although I have tried to define possibly unknown words throughout the text. Readers will know some of the words and phrases listed here, such as chronic fatigue syndrome.

Brain fog

Noticeable difficulty (to the individual and often to others) in which the person has trouble with thinking, concentrating, and remembering. Without treatment, brain fog is a common problem for people with chronic fatigue syndrome.

Chronic fatigue syndrome

A condition characterized by a significant decrease in the person's occupational, educational, social, or personal activities that persists for more than six months and is accompanied by fatigue, post-exertional malaise, and unrefreshing sleep. In addition, either cognitive impairment or orthostatic intolerance (or both conditions) is present.

Cognition

The ability to think clearly, express oneself to others, and concentrate. Without treatment, cognition may be impaired in people with chronic fatigue syndrome.

Dementia

A neurological disorder that impedes thinking and behavior. The most commonly known form of dementia is Alzheimer's disease.

Dopamine

A neurotransmitter that affects mood and behavior. Patients with depression may be prescribed antidepressants that boost dopamine levels.

Fibromyalgia

A painful chronic muscular condition that often presents along with chronic fatigue syndrome.

Hyperalgesia

An increased sensitivity to pain.

Lyme disease

An illness caused by a bite from the tick hosting the *Borrelia burgdorferi* bacterium. When diagnosing chronic fatigue syndrome, doctors may wish to rule out Lyme disease as well as other diseases such as fibromyalgia or multiple sclerosis.

Multiple sclerosis (MS)

A serious chronic inflammatory and neurodegenerative disease characterized by vision loss, pain, fatigue, and impaired coordination. Doctors may wish to rule out MS before diagnosing chronic fatigue syndrome.

Myalgic encephalomyelitis/chronic fatigue disorder (ME/CFS)

Two old diagnoses that are now used together to connote chronic fatigue syndrome.

Off-label prescribing

When a physician prescribes a medication that is not the FDA-approved indication for the drug. This is lawful and common, but the doctor should tell the patient why the medication is being prescribed and that it is being prescribed off-label.

Orthostatic intolerance/hypotension

A feeling of dizziness or imbalance that occurs after a person suddenly changes position from lying down to sitting up or from sitting to standing. Many people (but not all) with chronic fatigue syndrome experience this issue.

Placebo effect

A condition seen in clinical studies in which researchers give one group a medication and the other group a look-alike tablet or capsule that contains no medication. The group that does not receive the medication often believes they received the real drug and may report positive or negative effects. Researchers are very familiar with this phenomenon.

Postexertional malaise (PEM)

Severe exhaustion that may occur in a person with chronic fatigue syndrome after greater-than-usual physical or mental concentration. This condition occurs in most people with chronic fatigue syndrome when they extend themselves beyond their normal behavior.

Post-treatment Lyme disease syndrome

Symptoms of pain, fatigue, and brain fog that occur long after treatment with antibiotics.

Prescribed stimulants

Medications that may decrease fatigue, improve brain fog, and cut back on the pain levels in a person with chronic fatigue syndrome.

Prodrug

A drug that is converted to an active medication once it transfers from the gut into the bloodstream. This prodrug mechanism allows for a long-acting effect. Vyvanse is a prodrug.

Racemic mixture

When *dextro*-amphetamine and *levo*-amphetamine are combined in equal proportions in an amphetamine medication.

Restless legs syndrome

A disorder in which the sufferer has a compelling sensation to move about when lying down. The sensations may feel like an aching or a creeping feeling and are primarily experienced in the legs, but they may also occur in the arms or even the head or chest.

Serotonin

A neurotransmitter that affects mood and behavior. Sometimes people with depression are treated with antidepressants that boost serotonin levels, thus improving mood.

Sleep apnea

A condition characterized by short periods of breathing cessation during sleep. With this condition, the person periodically stops breathing for short periods. This condition requires treatment.

Systemic exertion intolerance disease (SEID)

Another name for chronic fatigue syndrome.

Wakefulness medications

Drugs that improve fatigue for people with narcolepsy and other disorders, sometimes used to treat the fatigue of chronic fatigue syndrome. Modafinil (Provigil) is the most common of these medications.

Appendix C: Screening Measures

In this appendix, I include information on three screening measures that psychiatrists and other physicians use to help them evaluate their patients. First are two fatigue measures, including the Fatigue Severity Scale (FSS) and the Fatigue Symptom Inventory. These two screening measures are often used in clinical studies.

- The Fatigue Severity Scale may be found online at this site: https://www.healthywomen.org/sites/default/files/FatigueSeverityScale.pdf
- The Fatigue Symptom Inventory is located at this site: http://www.cas.usf.edu/~jacobsen/FSI%20English%20Version.pdf
- The Patient Health Questionnaire (PHQ-9) was originally developed by Dr. Robert L. Spitzer and colleagues and is available to print. This questionnaire, presented on the next page, helps doctors diagnose depression.

PATIENT HEALTH QUESTIONNAIRE-9 (PHQ-9)

Over the past 2 weeks, how often have you been bothered by any of the following problems? (Use "✓" to indicate your answer	Not at all	Several days	More than half the days	Nearly every day
1. Little interest or pleasure in doing things				
2. Feeling down, depressed, or hopeless				
3. Trouble falling or staying asleep, or sleeping too much				
4. Feeling tired or having little energy				
5. Poor appetite or overeating				
6. Feeling bad about yourself—or that you are a failure or have let yourself or your family down				
7. Trouble concentrating on things, such as reading the newspaper or watching television				
8. Moving or speaking so slowly that other people could have noticed? Or the opposite—being so fidgety or restless that you have been moving around a lot more than usual				
9. Thoughts that you would be better off dead or of hurting yourself in some way				

FOR OFFICE CODING	0	+	+	+
			= Total Score	_____

If you checked off any problems, how difficult have these problems made it for you to do your work, take care of things at home, or get along with other people?

Not difficult at all	Somewhat difficult	Very difficult	Extremely difficult
☐	☐	☐	☐

Note: Developed by Drs. Robert L. Spitzer, Janet B. W. Williams, and Kurt Kroenke and colleagues, with an educational grant from Pfizer Inc. No permission required to reproduce, translate, display, or distribute.

For further information, please visit this site: https://www.phq.screeners .com.

Bibliography

Adamec, Christine, *Understanding Drugs: Amphetamines & Methamphetamine*. New York: Chelsea House, 2011.

Alltucker, Ken, "Marijuana as a Cure for Opioid Use? Nation's Top Drug Scientists Says She's Skeptical," *USA Today*, March 20, 2019, https://www.usatoday.com/story/news/health/2019/03/20/weed-marijuana-cannabis-opioid-addiction-withdrawal-nida-nora-volkow/3221792002/ (accessed May 1, 2019).

Alzheimer's Association, "A Public Health Approach to Alzheimer's and Other Dementias: Module 2: Alzheimer's and Other Dementias—The Basics," 2016, https://www.cdc.gov/aging/aginginfo/pdfs/A-Public-Health-Approach-To-Alzheimers.pdf (accessed June 20, 2019).

Alzheimer's Association, *2019 Alzheimer's Disease Facts and Figures*. Chicago, IL: Alzheimer's Association, 2019, https://www.alz.org/media/Documents/alzheimers-facts-and-figures-2019-r.pdf (accessed June 20, 2019).

American College of Cardiology, "2017 Guideline for the Prevention, Detection, Evaluation, and Management of High Blood Pressure in Adults," *Journal of the American College of Cardiology* (September 2017), https://www.acc.org/~/media/Non-Clinical/Files-PDFs-Excel-MS-Word-etc/Guidelines/2017/Guidelines_Made_Simple_2017_HBP.pdf (accessed August 22, 2019).

American Migraine Foundation, "Chronic Migraine," May 2008, https://americanmigrainefoundation.org/resource-library/chronic-migraine/ (accessed February 1, 2019).

American Sleep Apnea Association, "A Very Short Course on Sleep Apnea," n.d., https://www.sleepapnea.org/learn/sleep-apnea-information -clinicians/ (accessed June 12, 2019).

Ankar, Alex, and Kumar, Anil, "Vitamin B12 Deficiency (Cobalamin)," October 27, 2018, https://www.ncbi.nlm.nih.gov/books/NBK441923/ (accessed December 28, 2018).

Antshel, Kevin M., et al., "Posttraumatic Stress Disorder in Adult Attention-Deficit/Hyperactivity Disorder: Clinical Features and Familial Transmission," *Journal of Clinical Psychiatry* 74, n. 3 (2013): e197–e204.

Arria, Amelia M., et al., "Do College Students Improve Their Grades by Using Prescription Stimulants Nonmedically?" *Addictive Behavior* 65 (February 2017): 245–249.

Aviram, J., and Samuelly-Leichtag, G., "Efficacy of Cannabis-Based Medicines for Pain Management: A Systematic Review and Meta-Analysis of Randomized Controlled Trials," *Pain Physician* 21, n. 1 (2018): E79–E80. https://www.painphysicianjournal.com/current/pdf ?article=NDYwNA%3D%3D&journal=107 (accessed March 22, 2019).

Ballu, Pradeep C., and Kaur, Harleen, "Sleep Medicine: Insomnia and Sleep," *Missouri Medicine* 116, n. 1 (January/February 2019): 68–75.

Baumforth, K.R.N., et al., "The Epstein-Barr Virus and Its Association with Human Cancers," *Molecular Pathology* 52, n. 6 (December 1999): 307–322.

Bested, Alison C., and Marshall, Lynn M., "An Evidence-Based Approach to Diagnosis and Management by Clinicians," *Reviews on Environmental Health* 30, n. 4 (2015): 223–249.

Bested, Alison C., and Marshall, Lynn M., "Review of Myalgic Encephalomyelitis/Chronic Fatigue Syndrome," July 12, 2018, https://www .cdc.gov/me-cfs/about/possible-causes.html (accessed February 4, 2019).

Blockmans, Daniel, et al., "Does Methylphenidate Reduce the Symptoms of Chronic Fatigue Syndrome," *American Journal of Medicine* 119, n. 2 (February 2006): 167e23–167e30.

Boneva, Roumiana S., Lin, Jin-Mann S., and Unger, Elizabeth R., "Early Menopause and Other Gynecologic Risk Indicators for Chronic Fatigue Disease in Women," *Menopause* 22, n. 8 (August 2015): 826–834.

Bonn-Miller, Marcel O., et al., "Research Letter: Labeling Accuracy of Cannabidiol Extracts Sold Online," *Journal of the American Medical Association* 318, n. 2 (November 7, 2017): 1708–1709.

Bradley, N.G., and O'Brien, Angela, "Beyond ADHD and Narcolepsy: Psychostimulants in General Psychiatry," *Advances in Psychiatric Treatment* 15 (2009): 297–305.

Bransfield, Robert C., "Potential Uses of Modafinil in Psychiatric Disorders," *Journal of Applied Research* 4, n. 1 (2004): 198–207.

Brown, Molly M., and Jason, Leonard A., "Functioning in Individuals with Chronic Fatigue Syndrome: Increased Impairment with co-Occurring Multiple Chemical Sensitivity and Fibromyalgia," *Dynamic Medicine*, May 31, 2007, https://www.ncbi.nlm.nih.gov/pmc/articles/PMC1890280/pdf/1476-5918-6-6.pdf (accessed May 12, 2019).

Cassidy, Theresa A., et al., "Nonmedical Use and Diversion of ADHD Stimulants among U.S. Adults Ages 18–49: A National Internet Study," *Journal of Attention Disorders* 19, n. 7 (July 2015): 630–640.

Centers for Disease Control and Prevention, "Data and Surveillance: Lyme Disease," November 2, 2018, https://www.cdc.gov/lyme/data surveillance/index.html (accessed December 18, 2018).

Centers for Disease Control and Prevention, "Fibromyalgia," October 11, 2017, https://www.cdc.gov/arthritis/basics/fibromyalgia.htm (accessed February 1, 2019).

Centers for Disease Control and Prevention, "1 in 3 Adults Don't Get Enough Sleep," February 16, 2016, https://www.cdc.gov/media/releases/2016/p0215-enough-sleep.html (accessed June 16, 2019).

Centers for Disease Control and Prevention, "Possible Causes of Myalgic Encephalomyelitis/Chronic Fatigue Syndrome," n.d., https://www.cdc.gov/me-cfs/about/possible-causes.html (accessed May 10, 2019).

Centers for Disease Control and Prevention, "Primary Symptoms," n.d., https://www.cdc.gov.me-cfs/symptoms-diagnosis/symptoms.html (accessed December 31, 2018).

Centers for Disease Control and Prevention, "Signs and Symptoms of Untreated Lyme Disease," October 26, 2016, https://www.cdc.gov/lyme/signs_symptoms/index.html (accessed December 17, 2018).

Centers for Disease Control and Prevention, "Treatment," December 1, 2017, https://www.cdc.gov/lyme/treatment/index.html (accessed December 17, 2018).

Chandra, Jasvinder, "Insomnia," Medscape, September 11, 2018, https://emedicine.medscape.com/article/1187829-print (accessed June 12, 2019).

Chu, Lily, et al. "Deconstructing Post-Exertional Malaise in Myalgic Encephalomyelitis/Chronic Fatigue Syndrome: A Patient-Centered, Cross-Sectional Survey," *PLOS One* (June 1, 2018), https://doi.org/10.1371/journal.pone.0197811 (accessed December 31, 2018).

Committee on the Diagnostic Criteria for Myalgic Encephalomyelitis/ Chronic Fatigue Syndrome, Institute of Medicine of the National Academies, *Beyond Myalgic Encephalomyelitis/Chronic Fatigue Syndrome: Redefining an Illness*. Washington, DC: National Academies Press, 2015.

Concussion Legacy Foundation, "What Is CTE?" n.d., https://concussion foundation.org/CTE-resources/what-is-CTE (accessed June 20, 2019).

Daniels, Jo, Brigden, Amberly, and Kacorova, Adela, "Anxiety and Depression in Chronic Fatigue Syndrome/Myalgic Encephalomyelitis (CFS/ME): Examining the Incidence of Health Anxiety in CFS/ME," *Psychology and Psychotherapy: Theory, Research and Practice* (2017), https://onlinelibrary.wiley.com/doi/abs/10.1111/papt.12118 (accessed February 1, 2019).

Dilokthornsakul, Piyameth, et al., "Multiple Sclerosis Prevalence in the United States Commercially Insured Population," *Neurology* 86 (March 15, 2016): 1014–1021.

Eisen, Seth A., et al. "Gulf War Veterans' Health: Medical Evaluation of a U.S. Cohort," *Annals of Internal Medicine* 41 (2005): 881–890.

Fales, Jessica L., Ladd, Benjamin O., and Magnan, Renee E., "Pain Relief as a Motivation for Cannabis Use among Young Adult Users with and without Chronic Pain," *Journal of Pain* (2019), https://doi.org/1016/j .pain.2019.02.001 (accessed April 30, 2019).

Fernandez-de-las Penas, César, and Svensson, Peter. "Myofascial Temporomandibular Disorder," *Current Rheumatology Reviews* 12, n. 1 (2016): 40–54.

Fuller-Thomson, Esme, and Nimigon, Jodie, "Factors Associated with Depression among Individuals with Chronic Fatigue Syndrome: Findings from a Nationally Representative Study," *Family Practice Advance Access* (October 2008), https://academic.oup.com/fampra /article/25/6/414/480969 (accessed February 8, 2019).

Gadalla, T., "Association of Comorbid Mood Disorders and Chronic Illness with Disability and Quality of Life in Ontario, Canada," *Chronic Diseases in Canada* 28, n. 4 (2008): 148–154.

Gauer, Robert L., and Semidey, Michael J., "Diagnosis and Treatment of Temporomandibular Disorders," *American Family Physician* 91, n. 6 (May 15, 2015): 378–386.

Giloteaux, Ludovic, et al., "Reduced Diversity and Altered Composition of the Gut Microbiome in Individuals with Myalgic Encephalomyelitis/Chronic Fatigue Syndrome," *Microbiome* 4 (2016): 4–30.

Godman, Heidi, "How Much Water Should You Drink?" Harvard Health Publishing, July 18, 2018, https://www.health.harvard.edu

/staying-healthy/how-much-water-should-you-drink (accessed July 25, 2019).

Goss, Alexander J., et al., "Modafinil Augmentation Therapy in Unipolar and Bipolar Depression: A Systematic Review and Meta-Analysis of Randomized Controlled Trials," *Journal of Clinical Psychiatry* 74, n. 11 (November 2013): 1101–1107.

Grady, Denise, "Is a Virus the Cause of Fatigue Syndrome?" *New York Times*, October 12, 2009, https://www.nytimes.com/2009/10/13/health/13fatigue.html?searchresultPosition=8 (accessed October 1, 2019).

Grinspoon, Peter, "Cannabidiol (CBD)—What We Know and What We Don't," Harvard Health blog, Harvard Medical School, August 24, 2018, https://www.health.harvard.edu/blog/cannabidiol-cbd-what-we-know-and-what-we-dont-2018082414476 (accessed May 2, 2019).

Hande, Karen, "Cannabidiol," *Supportive Care* 23, n. 2 (April 2019): 131–134.

Heim, Christine, et al., "Early Adverse Experience and Risk for Chronic Fatigue Syndrome: Results from a Population-Based Study," *Archives of General Psychiatry* 66, n. 1 (January 2009): 72–80.

Ipaktchian, Susan, "14 Drugs Identified as Most Urgently Needing Study for Off-Label Use," Stanford University News Center, November 24, 2008, https://med.stanford.edu/news/all-news/2008/11/14-drugs-identified-as-most-urgently-needing-study-for-off-label-use-stanford-professor-says.html (accessed August 6, 2019).

Jain, Vageesh, et al., "Prevalence of and Risk Factors for Severe Cognitive and Sleep Symptoms in ME/CFS and MS," *BMC Neurology* 17 (2017), https://bmcneurol.biomedcentral.com/articles/10.1186/s12883-017-0896-0 (accessed February 2, 2018).

Johnson, Hillary, "Chasing the Shadow Virus," *Discover*, March 27, 2013, http://discovermagazine.com/2013/march/17-shadow-vir (accessed February 21, 2018).

Johnston, Samantha C., Staines, Donald R., and Marshall-Gradisnik, Sonya M., "Epidemiological Characteristics of Chronic Fatigue Syndrome/Myalgic Encephalomyelitis in Australian Patients," *Clinical Epidemiology* 8 (2016): 97–107.

Kallestad, Havard, et al., "The Role of Insomnia in the Treatment of Chronic Fatigue," *Journal of Psychosomatic Research* 78 (2015): 427–432.

Kandel, Joseph, and Sudderth, David, *The Headache Cure: How to Uncover What's Really Causing Your Pain and Find Lasting Relief.* New York: McGraw-Hill, 2006.

Kaser, Muzaffer, et al., "Modafinil Improves Episodic Memory and Working Memory Cognition in Patients with Remitted Depression: A Double-Blind, Randomized, Placebo-Controlled Study," *Biological Psychiatry: Cognitive Neuroscience and Neuroimaging* 2, n. 2 (2017): 115–122.

Kerr, Jonathan R. "Epstein-Barr Virus Induced Gene-2 Upregulation identifies a Particular Subtype of Chronic Fatigue Syndrome/Myalgic Encephalomyelitis," *Frontiers in Pediatrics* 7, n. 59 (March 2019): 1–11, https://www.ncbi.nlm.nih.gov/pmc/articles/PMC6424 879/ (accessed May 11, 2019).

Kingdon, Caroline C., et al., "Functional Status and Well-Being in People with Myalgic Encephalomyelitis/Chronic Fatigue Syndrome Compared with People with Multiple Sclerosis and Healthy Controls," *PharmacoEconomics Open* 2 (2018): 381–392.

Konuk, Numan, et al., "Open-Label Study of Adjunct Modafinil for the Treatment of Patients with Fatigue, Sleepiness, and Major Depression Treated with Selective Serotonin Reuptake Inhibitors," *Advances in Therapy* 23, n. 4 (July/August 2006): 646–654.

Leo, Raphael J., and Khalid, Kiren, "Antidepressants for Chronic Pain," *Current Psychiatry* 18, n. 2 (February 2019): 9–22.

Lin, Jin-Mann S., et al., "The Economic Impact of Chronic Fatigue Syndrome in Georgia: Direct and Indirect Costs," *Cost Effectiveness and Resource Allocation* 9, n. 1 (2011), https://link.springer.com/content /pdf/10.1186%2F1478-7547-9-1.pdf (accessed March 4, 2019).

Litleskare, S., et al., "Prevalence of Irritable Bowel Syndrome and Chronic Fatigue 10 Years after Giardia Infection," *Clinical Gastroenterology and Hepatology* 16, n. 7 (July 25, 2018):1064–1072.

Mayo Clinic, "Chronic Traumatic Encephalopathy," June 4, 2019, https://www.mayoclinic.org/diseases-conditions/chronic-traumatic -encephalopathy/symptoms-causes/syc-20370921 (accessed June 20, 2019).

McFadden, Robert D., "Frances Oldham Kelsey, Who Saved U.S. Babies from Thalidomide, Dies at 101," *New York Times*, August 7, 2015, https://www.nytimes.com/2015/08/08/science/frances-oldham-kelsey -fda-doctor-who-exposed-danger-of-thalidomide-dies-at-101.html (accessed May 2, 2019).

The MTA Cooperative Group Multimodal Treatment of Children with ADHD, "A 14-Month Randomized Clinical Trial of Treatment Strategies for Attention Deficit/Hyperactivity Disorder," *Archives of General Psychiatry* 56, n. 12 (December 1999): 1973–1086.

Murphy, Gwen, et al., "Meta-Analysis Shows That Prevalence of Epstein-Barr Virus-Positive Gastric Cancer Differs Based on Sex and Anatomic Location," *Gastroenterology* 137, n. 3 (September 2009): 824–833.

National Academies of Sciences, Engineering, and Medicine. *The Health Effects of Cannabis and Cannabinoids: The Current States of Evidence and Recommendations for Research.* Washington, DC: The National Academies Press, 2017, page 90.

National Center for Complementary and Integrative Health, "Lyme Disease," March 2019, https://www.nccih.nih.gov/health/lyme-disease (accessed April 17, 2020).

National Conference of State Legislatures, "Drugged Driving/Marijuana-Impaired Driving," March 8, 2019, http://www.ncsl.org/research/transportation/drugged-driving-overview.aspx (accessed March 22, 2019).

National Conference of State Legislatures, "State Medical Marijuana Laws," March 5, 2019, http://www.ncsl.org/research/health/state-medical-marijuana-laws.aspx (accessed March 22, 2019).

National Headache Foundation, "Illness, Chronic Fatigue Syndrome and Migraine," March 15, 2013, https://headaches.org/2013/09/15/illness-chronic-fatigue-syndrome-and-migraine/ (accessed February 7, 2019).

National Institute of Mental Health, "Generalized Anxiety Disorder," November 2017, https://www.nimh.nih.gov/health/statistics/generalized-anxiety-disorder.shtml (accessed February 1, 2019).

National Institute of Mental Health, "Major Depression," November 2017, https://www.nimh.nih.gov/health/statistics/major-depression.shtml (accessed February 1, 2019).

National Institute of Neurological Disorders and Stroke, "Restless Legs Syndrome Fact Sheet," May 2017, https://www.ninds.nih.gov/disorders/patient-caregiver-education/fact-sheets/restless-legs-syndrome-fact-sheet (accessed June 16, 2019).

National Institute on Deafness and Other Communications Disorders, "Tinnitus," March 6, 2017, https://www.nidcd.nih.gov/health/tinnitus (accessed February 7, 2019).

National Institutes of Health, "Magnesium," September 26, 2018, https://ods.od.nih.gov/factsheets/magnesium-HealthProfessional/ (accessed December 26, 2019).

National Institutes of Health, Office of Dietary Supplements, "Vitamin B12: Fact Sheet for Health Professionals," November 29, 2018, https://ods.od.nih.gov/factsheets/vitaminb12-HealthProfessional/ (accessed December 17, 2018).

National Multiple Sclerosis Society, "Fatigue," n.d., https://www
.nationalmssociety.org/Symptoms-Diagnosis/MS-Symptoms/Fatigue
(accessed December 17, 2018).

Nayak, M., and Bhattacharyya, P.C., "Chronic Fatigue Syndrome,"
Journal of Evidence Based Medicine and Healthcare 4, n. 88 (2017):
5213–5217, https://doi.org/10.18410/jebmh/2017/1041.

Nelson, Harry, *The United States of Opioids: A Prescription for Liberating a Nation in Pain.* New York: ForbesBooks, 2019.

Noonan, Curtis W., et al., "The Prevalence of Multiple Sclerosis in 3 US
Communities," *Preventing Chronic Disease* 7, n. 1 (January 2010),
https://www.ncbi.nlm.nih.gov/pmc/articles/PMC2811507/ (accessed
December 28, 2018).

Norman, James, "Hypothyroidism: Overview, Causes, and Symptoms,"
Endocrineweb, November 27, 2018, https://www.endocrineweb
.com/conditions/thyroid/hypothyroidism-too-little-thyroid-hormone
(accessed December 28, 2018).

Novak, Scott P., et al., "The Nonmedical Use of Prescription ADHD
Medications: Results from a National Panel," *Substance Abuse
Treatment, Prevention, and Policy,* October 2007, https://substance
abusepolicy.biomedcentral.com/track/pdf/10.1186/1747-597X-2-32
(accessed August 13, 2019).

Ocon, Anthon J., "Caught in the Thickness of Brain Fog: Exploring
the Cognitive Symptoms of Chronic Fatigue Syndrome," *Frontiers in
Physiology* 4, n. 63 (April 2013), https://www.ncbi.nlm.nih.gov/pmc
/articles/PMC3617392/pdf/fphys-04-00063.pdf (accessed May 22,
2019).

Office on Women's Health, "Bladder Pain," December 27, 2018, https://
www.womenshealth.gov/a-z-topics/bladder-pain (accessed February
7, 2019).

Office on Women's Health, "Fibromyalgia," August 22, 2017, https://
www.womenshealth.gov/files/documents/fact-sheet-fibromyalgia.pdf
(accessed February 7, 2019).

Office of Women's Health, "Insomnia," November 30, 2017, https://
www.womenshealth.gov/a-z-topics/insomnia (accessed June 10,
2019).

Ohler, Norman, *Blitzed: Drugs in Nazi Germany.* New York: Penguin
Press, 2017.

Olson, L.G., Ambrogetti, A., and Sutherland, D.C., "A Pilot Randomized
Controlled Trial of Dexamphetamine in Patients with Chronic Fatigue
Syndrome," *Psychosomatics* 44, n. 1 (January–February 2003): 38–43.

O'Souza, Deepak Cyril, and Ranganathan, Mohini, "Medical Marijuana: Is the Cart before the Horse?" *Journal of the American Medical Association* 313, n. 24 (June 23–30, 2015): 2431–2432.

Park, Kyung Mee, et al., "Cognitive Behavioral Therapy for Insomnia Reduces Hypnotic Prescriptions," *Psychiatry Investigation* (2017), https://www.ncbi.nlm.nih.gov/pmc/articles/PMC5976005/pdf/pi -2017-11-20.pdf (accessed June 10, 2019).

Parker, Romy, et al., "The Effects of Warm Water Immersion on Blood Pressure, Heart Rate and Heart Rate Variability in People with Chronic Fatigue Syndrome," *South African Journal of Physiotherapy* 74, n. 1 (August 2018), https://www.ncbi.nlm.nih.gov/pmc/articles /PMC6131699/pdf/SAJP-74-442.pdf (accessed July 24, 2019).

Prior, Ryan, "He Pioneered Technology that Fueled the Human Genome Project. Now His Greatest Challenge Is Curing His Own Son," CNN, https://www.cnn.com/2019/05/12/health/stanford-geneticist-chronic -fatigue-syndrome-trnd/index.html (accessed May 13, 2019).

Reynolds, Kenneth J., et al., "The Economic Impact of Chronic Fatigue Syndrome," *Cost Effectiveness and Resource Allocation* (2004), https:// resource-allocation.biomedcentral.com/track/pdf/10.1186/1478 -7547-2-4 (accessed March 8, 2019).

Rimes, Katharine A., et al., "Emotional Suppression in Chronic Fatigue Syndrome: Experimental Study," *Health Psychology* 35, n. 9 (2016): 979–986.

Russell, Alice, et al., "Persistent Fatigue Induced by Interferon-Alpha: A Novel, Inflammation-Based, Proxy Model of Chronic Fatigue Syndrome," *Psychoneuroendocrinology* (December 17, 2018), https://reader .elsevier.com/reader/sd/pii/S0306453018301963 (accessed December 18, 2018).

Sáez-Francás, Naia, et al., "Attention-Deficit Hyperactivity Disorder in Chronic Fatigue Syndrome Patients," *Psychiatry Research* 200 (2012): 748–753.

Schmaling, Karen B., and Betterton, Karran L., "Neurocognitive Complaints and Functional Status among Patients with Chronic Fatigue Syndrome and Fibromyalgia," *Quality Life Research* 25, n. 5 (May 2016): 1257–1263.

Schrot, Richard J., and Hubbard, John R., "Cannabinoids: Medical Implications," *Annals of Medicine* 48, n. 3 (2016): 128–141.

Stephen M. Stahl, *Stahl's Essential Psychopharmacology Prescriber's Guide. Sixth Edition.* Cambridge, UK: Cambridge University Press, 2017.

Strawn, Jeffrey R., and Picard, Lara S., "Triple-Bead Mixed Amphetamine Salt for ADHD," *Current Psychiatry* 16, n. 8 (August 2017): 33–37.

Turkington, Douglas, et al., "Recovery from Chronic Fatigue Syndrome with Modafinil," *Human Psychopharmacology Clinical and Experimental* 19 (2004): 63–64.

Underhill, R.A., "Myalgic Encephalomyelitis, Chronic Fatigue Syndrome: An Infectious Disease," *Medical Hypotheses* 85 (2015): 765–773.

Unger, Elizabeth R., et al., "CDC Grand Rounds: Chronic Fatigue Syndrome—Advancing Research and Clinical Education," *Morbidity and Mortality Weekly* 65, n. 50–51 (December 2016): 1434–1438.

van Campen, C.M.C., Rowe, P.C., and Visser, F.C., "Blood Volume Status in ME/CFA Correlates with Presence or Absence of Orthostatic Symptoms: Preliminary Results." *Frontiers in Pediatrics* 6 (November 15, 2018), https://www.frontiersin.org/articles/10.3389/fped.2018.00352 /full (accessed March 16, 2020).

Veterans Administration, "Chronic Fatigue Syndrome in Gulf War Veterans," December 27, 2017, https://www.publichealth.va.gov/exposures /gulfwar/chronic-fatigue-syndrome.asp (accessed February 13, 2018).

Veterans Administration, "Fibromyalgia in Gulf War Veterans," December 27, 2017, https://www.publichealth.va.gov/exposures/gulfwar /fibromyalgia.asp (accessed February 13, 2018).

Veterans Administration Employment Toolkit, "Relaxation Exercise: Progressive Muscle Relaxation," n.d., https://www.va.gov/vetsinwork place/docs/em_eap_exercise_PMR.asp (accessed June 10, 2019).

Viner, Russell, and Hotopf, Matthew, "Childhood Predictors of Self-Reported Chronic Fatigue Syndrome/Myalgic Encephalomyelitis in Adults: National Birth Cohort Study," *British Medical Journal* (October 6, 2004), https://www.ncbi.nlm.nih.gov/pmc/articles/PMC524102 /pdf/bmj32900941.pdf (accessed February 4, 2019).

Warner, M.J., and Kamran, M.T., "Anemia, Iron Deficiency," November 14, 2018, https://www.ncbi.nlm.nih.gov/books/NBK448065/ (accessed December 18, 2018).

Whiteside, Alan, Hansen, Stig, and Chaudhuri, Abhijit, "Exercise Lowers Pain Threshold in Chronic Fatigue Syndrome," *Pain* 109 (2004): 497–499.

Whiting, Penny F., et al., "Cannabinoids for Medical Use: A Systematic Review and Meta-Analysis," *Journal of the American Medical Association* 313, n. 24 (2015): 2456–2473.

Wiffen, Philip J., Derry, Sheena, and Moore, R. Andrew, "Lamotrigine for Acute and Chronic Pain," *Cochrane Database Systems Review* (2011),

https://www.cochranelibrary.com/cdsr/doi/10.1002/14651858.CD0
06044.pub3/epdf/full (accessed May 1, 2019).

Woznicki, Katrina, "FDA Approves Cymbalta for Chronic Musculo-skeletal Pain," November 5, 2010, https://www.webmd.com/pain
-management/news/20101105/fda-approves-cymbalta-for-chronic
-musculoskeletal-pain (accessed July 11, 2019).

Young, Joel, "ADHD Is Notable Characteristic of Patients Suffering
from Chronic Lyme Disease: A Survey of Adults at the Michigan
Lyme Disease Association Conference," American Psychiatric Asso-ciation Annual Meeting, Philadelphia, PA, May 4, 2012, NRD-30,
p. 212, https://borderlinepersonalitydisorder.org/wp-content/uploads
/2012/04/2012_apa_program_guide1.pdf (accessed May 5, 2019.)

Young, Joel L., "Use of Lisdexamfetamine Dimesylate in Treatment of
Executive Functioning Deficits and Chronic Fatigue Syndrome: A
Double Blind, Placebo-Controlled Study," *Psychiatry Research* 207
(2013): 127–133.

Index

About the Author

Joel L. Young, MD, is the medical director and founder of the Rochester Center for Behavioral Medicine in Rochester Hills, Michigan. Dr. Young is certified by the American Board of Psychiatry and Neurology with added qualifications in geriatric, forensic, and adolescent psychiatry. In addition, he serves as a Clinical Associate Professor of Psychiatry at the Wayne State University School of Medicine. Dr. Young is Chief Medical Officer of the Clinical Trials Group of Southeast Michigan, where he has served as primary investigator for more than 90 clinical trials. He has authored many articles on psychiatric issues and several books, including *ADHD Grown Up: A Guide to Adolescent and Adult ADHD* (2007), *Contemporary Guide to Adult ADHD* (2009), and *When Your Adult Child Breaks Your Heart: Coping with Mental Illness, Substance Abuse, and the Problems That Tear Families Apart* (2013). He lives with his wife and two golden retrievers in Bloomfield Hills, Michigan. He relishes time with his adult children. For decades Dr. Young has championed the cause that fatigue is a common and profoundly debilitating symptom, often minimized by medical professionals. This book represents a sustained project, anchored by his own clinical research, to offer patients and practitioners hope in the treatment of chronic fatigue syndrome.